Care of the
Nursing-Home Patient

CARE OF THE NURSING-HOME PATIENT

———◆•◆———

EDITED BY

Langdon Hooper, M.D.

SOMETIME ASSISTANT PROFESSOR OF MEDICINE
YALE UNIVERSITY SCHOOL OF MEDICINE
NEW HAVEN
FORMERLY CHIEF, HOSPITAL SECTION, CONNECTICUT STATE
DEPARTMENT OF HEALTH
HARTFORD

AND

Paul A. McWilliams

ASSOCIATE DIRECTOR, MC GREGOR MEMORIAL CONFERENCE CENTER
WAYNE STATE UNIVERSITY
DETROIT, MICHIGAN
FORMERLY ASSISTANT DIRECTOR, CONTINUING EDUCATION
UNIVERSITY OF CONNECTICUT
STORRS, CONNECTICUT

———◆•◆———

LITTLE, BROWN AND COMPANY
BOSTON

PRINTED IN THE UNITED STATES OF AMERICA

Preface

PROFESSIONAL workers concerned with the care of patients in nursing homes have raised many questions about the quality of present-day programs. The content and responsibilities of this relatively new type of medical-care facility are still being defined: the need for more medical and nursing supervision is apparent; an understanding of the nutritional requirements of the patient is necessary; the reasons for cleanliness both of the patient and the home must be appreciated; the provision of sound rehabilitation programs is a concern of all.

This text has been prepared in order to discuss some of these issues and in the hope that it will serve as an information source and a guide for the many professional persons now staffing nursing homes. The material presented was developed from courses given to supervising nurses in nursing homes; it also reflects the professional experience of specialists in medicine, psychiatry, pharmacology, bacteriology, rehabilitation, and other fields.

The editors thank the nurse consultants of the Hospital Section of the Connecticut State Department of Health as well as Mrs. Dorothy Mullen, Mrs. Marion Zetterstom, Miss Charlotte Smith, and Miss Mary Bracket for their assistance with source material. We are also grateful for the editorial assistance of Mr. Howland Porter Hall of the publisher's staff.

This work has been partially supported by United States Public Health Service Grant No. S.T.T.-144-64(CH).

L. H.

P. A. McW.

Contributing Authors

William Baird, M.D.
Chief, Intermediate Service
Veterans Administration Hospital, West Haven, Connecticut

John Donnelly, M.D.
Psychiatrist-in-Chief, Institute of Living, Hartford, Connecticut

David S. Fischer, M.D.
Assistant Clinical Professor of Medicine
Yale University School of Medicine, New Haven, Connecticut

Ruth B. Kundsin, Sc.D.
Assistant in Surgery
Peter Bent Brigham Hospital, Boston, Massachusetts

William G. Leeds, M.D.
Attending Physician, Hartford Hospital, Hartford, Connecticut

vii

Contributing Authors

Raymond M. Massengill, Jr., M.S.
Director, Medical Speech Pathology
Duke University Medical Center, Durham, North Carolina

William Prestley, M.D.
Attending Physician, Hartford Hospital, Hartford, Connecticut

Contents

———•••———

Care of the
Nursing-Home Patient

1

Background and
Development

———◆•◆———

N U R S I N G homes are widely recognized as having a
significant role in the total medical-care program. The
recent expansion in both the number and size of nursing
homes, particularly those supplying medical care of high
quality, has attracted the attention of the public and
the interest of professional groups. The importance of
the nursing home in the total medical-care program is
emphasized by its inclusion in the Medicare Act passed
by the United States Congress.

Evolution of the Nursing Home

The nursing home is a product not only of the tremendous achievements of medicine over the past 50
years, but also of the evolution of a rapidly developing
civilization. A century ago the elderly person who could
no longer care for himself had these alternatives: being
cared for by a relative or becoming the town's respon-

sibility. In the latter case, he was placed in 12 different homes annually, spending one month in each. The small payment received from the town by each home owner hardly covered the cost of food, much less of nursing care. Nursing homes and homes for the aged were almost nonexistent.

Since World War II especially, fewer and fewer families have been willing or able to take their elderly relatives into their homes. Houses are smaller, more and more housewives do outside work, many families move frequently, and there has been a growing understanding of what is best—not just possible—for the elderly. The increasing complexity of our society requires more and more participation by town, state, and federal governments to deal with social problems. Nursing homes of a custodial nature were the first to spring up; only in the last few years [comparatively recently] has the medical aspect of the nursing home been stressed.

Medical-care facilities involve medical-care practices, and it is largely because of the widespread advances in medicine that the nursing home has become a necessity. A century ago tuberculosis, typhoid fever, dysentery, diphtheria, and malaria were commonplace. For example, in 1885 in Bridgeport, Connecticut, then a small city of 35,000, there were 90 deaths from tuberculosis, 90 from dysentery in children under 5 years of age, 40 from diphtheria, and 5 from malaria. The toll of such diseases was accepted, as inevitable. From childhood, people were exposed to virulent epidemics and many children and adults succumbed. The short life span was a pattern. In the 1880s physicians and clinical investigators began to expand the knowledge of disease. The tubercule bacillus was isolated first, then the bacilli for typhoid and diphtheria. In the next few decades new methods to combat these infections developed. With each decade of advance the chance for survival increased, and the average life span was extended.

During the last fifty years, the contagious-disease hospital has disappeared, the number of beds in tuberculosis hospitals has been markedly reduced, and the general hospital for diagnosis and treatment has been widely accepted. Antibiotics and preventive programs have reduced mortality. Advances in surgical techniques, anesthesiology, and blood banks have also prolonged life. These factors and the constantly increasing numbers in the total population have brought about a marked increase in the group of 65 years of age. In the United States this number has grown from three million in 1900 to over eighteen million in 1965. It is anticipated that this trend will continue.

Some provision must be made for the care of this enlarged elderly population. The general hospitals do not have the bed capacity to care for all of the patients requiring care in a medical facility. Since the number of hospital beds has not kept pace with the increasing demand for services, access to the general hospital has become limited to the acutely ill and the short-term patient. Increasingly, the patient requiring a longer stay is transferred to other facilities. The nursing home is one such facility developed to provide necessary care for such patients.

The objectives, standards, and criteria for the nursing home have not yet been clearly defined, however. This has led to confusion concerning the proper operation of such homes. State authorities have therefore promulgated regulations governing the operation and maintenance of such facilities. In some states these have been placed under the supervision of the welfare departments because many of the patients and residents receive welfare aid. This comports with the concept that the nursing home is custodial in function and replaces the almshouse and county farm. Other state authorities approach the problem from its medical aspect: since nursing homes care for ill patients, rules and regulations governing their operation should be administered by the state department of health. The American Medical Association and the American Nursing Home Association have recently formed a joint committee to develop an accreditation program, but it will require time to reconcile the wide differences in concepts of standards in the 50 states and to develop acceptable and meaningful criteria.

Medical Problems of the Elderly

The nursing-home problem must be approached with an open mind, avoiding preconceptions. The medical, nursing, and social needs of patients with such disorders as arteriosclerosis, congestive heart failure, diabetes mellitus, fractures, and terminal cancer must be defined. *Functional capacity* as well as diagnosis must be considered in providing adequate medical and nursing care. Such classification of patients according to their needs has been developed for the Connecticut State Welfare Department.

A survey in Connecticut nursing homes was made to determine the diagnosis and the functional capacity of patients requiring institutional care. The largest group —55 per cent—consisted of patients with cardiovascular arteriosclerosis. Mental confusion, inability to dress, and incontinence were present in varying degrees, necessitating continual supervision and care. Severe cardiac cases—patients with decompensation and peripheral or pulmonary edema—accounted for 3.8 per cent. Fracture cases (6 per cent) were restricted to recent fractures of the hip or lower extremity or to nonunion of a fracture. The neurological cases (8.5 per cent) included multiple sclerosis, Parkinson's disease, and other disabling neurological diseases. Cancer patients listed (5 per cent) were those who had advanced or terminal cancer. Arthritis cases (2 per cent) included in the seriously ill group were those who had advanced disease and were severely restricted in their movements.

Types of Nursing Homes

Not all general hospitals offer all services to all patients; community hospitals offer limited services to patients when compared to the university or teaching hospital with services in all subspecialties. Similarly, one must not expect all nursing homes to provide all types of care for all patients. In Connecticut some nursing homes have many services available for the convalescent patient, while other homes with less seriously ill patients offer limited services.

Since 1955, many individuals and groups have become interested in the problems of nursing-home care, and from their interest and leadership have evolved a number of nursing homes with excellent programs for the care of both custodial and seriously ill patients. Nonprofit and voluntary organizations, including religious bodies, are participating in this area and have founded nursing homes that offer medical care. Some nonprofit homes, however, care for only a small proportion of elderly patients. The care for the largest number of such patients is provided by the proprietary nursing homes. Some of these are well supervised and offer high quality care; others do not have sufficient staff or facilities to provide adequate medical and nursing care to the seriously ill long-term patient.

Medicare and the Nursing Home

Legislation passed by the Eighty-ninth Congress in 1965 will be significant in the further growth and development of nursing homes. Public Law 89-97 (Medicare) provides for posthospital extended-care services for up to "one hundred days during any spell of illness in individuals over 65 years old." Payment will be made to those who provide such services at a reasonable cost, which is determined by the Secretary of Health, Education, and Welfare. Posthospital care applies to those who have been inpatients for not less than 3 consecutive days and who are admitted to the second institution within 14 days of hospital discharge.

The description of the extended-care facility follows the concept of an institution that provides medical rather than custodial care. The Medicare Act requires a written transfer agreement between the nursing home and a hospital. Patients are to be transferred when it is medically appropriate; there is also to be an exchange of medical information between the hospital and the nursing home. In order to ensure reasonable transfer of such patients, each hospital is to have a Utilization Committee comprised of two staff physicians and such additional personnel as may be necessary. Review will be made on admission regarding the duration of the patient's stay and the need for professional services. A regimen will be specified, and the individual, the physician, and the institution will be notified of the results of the review. The Utilization Committee may be formed by the local medical society and one or more hospitals.

The Medicare Act recognizes that extended care requires both skilled nursing and rehabilitative services. A policy is to be developed by one or more physicians and one or more registered nurses for patient care. A physician and a registered nurse are to be responsible for carrying out such policies for each patient. Clinical records are to be maintained on all patients; 24-hour nursing service is to be provided, with at least one registered professional nurse on duty at all times. Other requirements involve the specification of appropriate methods and procedures for dispensing and administering drugs and biologicals, and a utilization review plan.

The Eighty-ninth Congress also passed the Older Americans Act. This act combines governmental departments handling the affairs of the aged under one commissioner in the Department of Health, Education, and Welfare; he is appointed by the President with Senate approval. The act authorizes funds for grants to the states for five years for community planning demonstrations, training of personnel, and establishment of programs for the aging. It also authorizes grants to nonprofit organizations for research and development in this field. This legislation recognizes the changing population patterns in the country and the needs of the aging. It involves formal commitments to improve care in an area that has too long been ignored.

New paths are being explored, new approaches created, and new programs devised for the care of the elderly. Long-term care in a nursing home requires medical and nursing supervision which is very expensive. Medicare does not, however, cover all costs of such care. Insurance and other third-party payment companies have a responsibility to develop insurance plans for some classes of patients and some nursing homes. Definitions, standards, and costs need to be developed. The Hunterdon Medical Center at Flemington, New Jersey, has worked out such a plan with the New Jersey Blue Cross. Such plans must assume that there are or will be adequate and competent medical and nursing programs. Residents and patients have illnesses that are caused by disease processes, not just aging: they must receive competent advice, treatment and followup care. As such supplementary plans develop, they will make a special contribution to better patient care.

2
Staffing the Nursing Home

———◆•◆———

I T is increasingly recognized that the role of the nursing home is changing. Formerly it provided custodial
care to elderly persons, some of whom were ill enough
to be bedridden and thus required some nursing care.
By contrast, the nursing home of today is more and
more regarded as a medical-care facility that provides
skilled nursing care under medical supervision for the
chronically ill. Low-cost housing is provided by both
the state and the federal governments for elderly persons who are ambulatory and still able to care for themselves. Present-day nursing homes are thus faced with
the choice of either becoming homes for the elderly
offering purely custodial care, or gradually evolving into
true nursing homes that provide skilled nursing care.
The latter type of care cannot be provided unless the
home is suitably staffed and unless the staff and the
medical services are properly organized. This fact was
clearly recognized by the federal government when it

9

specified certain minimum staffing requirements in the Medicare Act.

The Medicare Act has set certain minimum requirements regarding the medical staffing of nursing homes. Every home is required to have a physician and a registered nurse who are responsible for medical, nursing, and rehabilitative policies. The home is required to have 24-hour nursing coverage. At present, few homes can fulfill these requirements. There is a shortage of nurses, and such staffing is expensive. With the passing of the Medicare Act, it is hoped that the general public will gradually become aware of the need for proper support for nursing homes. Since the majority of patients in nursing homes in the United States are receiving some welfare assistance, good care and adequate staffing can be achieved only by realistic welfare rates. Administrators and owners of good nursing homes must continue to educate the public and, particularly, their communities as to the service they provide. The general reputation of nursing homes is usually based on that of the substandard home. Much effort will be required to change this image.

Role of the Administrator

Nearly 90 per cent of all nursing homes are proprietary, and the owner is ultimately responsible for the type of home and the quality of care. The owner may be the administrator or he may hire an administrator to run the home. In either case the administrator should have knowledge of and experience concerning the care of the sick, preferably in a similar medical-care facility. He must recruit, supervise, and educate his staff.

One of the problems encountered in proprietary homes is the proper delegation of authority. Experience dictates that the responsibility for medical services must rest with the physician, not with the administrator or nursing staff. The owner or administrator may be unwilling to relinquish such authority, failing to realize that delegation of responsibility regarding medical matters to the physician or relegation of nursing techniques to the graduate nurse does not mean that he will lose control. Like the hospital administrator, the nursing-home administrator should set up and coordinate medical, nursing, dietary, housekeeping and other necessary departments. The more medically oriented these facilities become, the greater and more complex will be the administrative responsibilities, so that more authority must be delegated. The provision of the Medicare Act specifying transfer agreements with hospitals, for example, requires increased paperwork and greater coordination.

Therefore, proper staffing of the nursing home becomes one of the most important tasks of the administrator. He must obtain the services of a good physician and support him with a well-run nursing service, one headed by a registered nurse and able to carry out a medical program. If the quality of nursing is poor, physicians will lose interest in attending to the medical needs of the patients. If there is no physician-in-charge to provide a comprehensive and continuing medical program, skilled nurses will not be attracted to work in nursing homes.

Finally, the administrator does much to set the tone of a nursing home. His attitudes and reactions to the patients will usually carry over to the staff. If the administrator is concerned about the patient as an individual—for example, acting as a catalyst in stimulating the physician-in-charge, the nurses, and any paramedical personnel (such as part-time physical therapist working toward the rehabilitation of a stroke patient)—the morale of the entire nursing home will improve. If, on the other hand, he regards the patients only as a source of income and allows them merely to "exist" and not to "live," the general atmosphere will be one of depression and despair. Such an attitude is detrimental, not only to the patients but also to the staff, who would rather work in more pleasant and hopeful surroundings.

The Physician's Responsibility

Observation and experience indicate that, where there is good medical and nursing supervision, the patient's medical needs are met; where supervision is lacking, the program can be poor. Present regulations in many states and the Medicare Act itself require that a registered nurse supervise nursing care. In many nursing homes, because of the organization, nurses have been compelled to asume more responsibilities than their qualifications justify. Such practice should not be allowed to continue.

Some state regulations require that a physician visit the patient every 30 days; such regulations do not insure good care. A seriously ill patient may require daily visits; patients in a better condition may need to be examined only at two- to three-month intervals. This requires judgment based on clinical experience. Certainly, a registered nurse-supervisor does not wish to assume such responsibility. Some nursing homes have a medical staff organized like that of the general hospital. Although the existence of a staff so organized does not guarantee perfect care, experience indicates that patient care is improved when the medical staff is properly organized.

The physician-in-charge or a staff committee of physicians must supervise and be responsible for all medical care. A comprehensive medical program should be developed not only for each patient, but also for the nursing home as a whole. The physician and the administrator should come to an agreement as to who is responsible for the medical program, the organization of the medical personnel, and the responsibility within this chain of command on medical matters. If these questions can be settled at the outset, with continued close cooperation there can be a free interchange between doctor and nurse concerning medical care.

The Joint Commission on Accreditation of Hospitals discusses the duties and responsibilities of a chief of service for a department in a general hospital. It sets forth these general principles:

He is responsible for the proper management and quality of service in his department. He is responsible for enforcement of hospital bylaws, rules, and regulations with special attention to his department. He should be available for consultations in his field. He should cooperate with hospital administration in formulating special regulations and policies. He should check medical records. He is responsible for teaching and education in his department. He enforces consultation of services.

These general principles can also be applied to the physicians-in-charge in the nursing home. At present, for example, if a patient has been seen once, he may not be seen again for 30 days, following present state health and welfare regulations. In some homes patients have not seen a physician for as long as three to six months. The private physician is not subject to supervision, as he is in a general hospital. Thus, a physician appointed by the nursing home to supervise and assume responsibility for the medical needs of all patients—his duties being similar to those of the chief of a medical department—can raise the level of medical care. Once the quality of medical practice, and the need for additional visits and consultations have been delegated to him, it then becomes his responsibility to see that accepted practices and procedures are followed.

The physician-in-charge should visit the nursing home at least twice a week, although daily visits are preferable. The medical records of all patients should be reviewed periodically, with the nursing supervisor in attendance. Changes of treatment should be discussed with the nurse. Often the nursing supervisor can offer valuable information on a patient's condition, as on rounds in a general hospital. If a patient has his own physician, he should be made fully aware of his responsibility for medical visits to his patient. If the span between visits is too long, a reminder can be sent to the attending physician. This information can be kept on the patient's medical record.

Since the Medicare Act requires a written transfer agreement between the nursing home and a hospital, with exchange of information between the two, the services of the hospital and the nursing home should be coordinated. The hospital can provide laboratory, x-ray, and other diagnostic facilities, as well as consultation in nursing, diet, and physical and occupational therapy; in turn, the nursing home provides opportunities for teaching nursing care for the chronically ill and the geriatric patient. The physician and the administrator should work closely to establish an affiliation.

In New York City, the Department of Welfare has inaugurated several new arrangements with physicians to obtain better care for its clients in nursing homes. They include arrangements with a team of family physicians to provide the welfare patients with care, with an internist as overall director, and an agreement whereby a hospital, through its attending and resident staff, assumes responsibility for the complete medical care of a nearby nursing home's residents, both in the home and in the hospital. Experience has shown that, with such teams, fewer emergency trips to the hospital are required. These efforts are often supplemented by a social service worker. This approach, obtaining closer cooperation with the family physician and the hospital, is another means to improve the level of care.

MEDICAL RECORDS

The medical record is an integral part of patient care and is used to establish the diagnosis as well as to record the patient's course. The medical record is also used to measure the quality of work. Medical Audit Committees are common in many general hospitals. It is their duty to review all records to ascertain that accepted procedures have been followed and then report to the staff.

The medical record begins with the patient's history. Information is obtained on his present illness and, in orderly sequence, on all body systems. Questions are asked on previous illnesses that may apply to the present complaint. Some diagnoses are arrived at on the basis of a careful history alone. The physical examination follows, also with a check of all body systems. Laboratory work is then ordered, to supply supplementary data to assist in the diagnosis. The diagnosis is the result of all the information obtained from these three sources. The record continues with progress notes (which are recorded every three days) and consultation notes, as required. The nurse enters the patient's vital signs on the temperature sheet every four hours, as well as her notes recording the patient's general condition and the medications given.

Such detailed information is not necessary for all patients in the long-term care institution. Sufficient information should be provided, however, to justify the diagnosis and warrant continued treatment of the patient. Nursing regulations require that a medical record be kept for each patient; proper identification, physician's findings, diagnosis, and orders must be included, and the nurses must record all medications and the patient's condition each day. Since nursing-home residents will increasingly be medical patients requiring treatment for specific disease syndromes, it becomes the responsibility of the physician-in-charge to see that a complete and up-to-date record is maintained. The record, to be complete, should present orderly and accurate medical information necessary for the proper management and evaluation of the case. Simple recordings of the medical diagnosis or of a symptom complex does not constitute a medical record. A recommended form that has been widely accepted by nursing homes and physicians is shown in Figure 1.

The admission sheet is divided into four sections. The

ADMISSION RECORD

Full Name_____

Residence No. _____ Street_____ Town_____

Date of Admission___ AM__ PM__Date of Discharge ____ AM__PM__

Sex_____ Race_____ Religion_____

Date of Birth (year, month, day) _____

Single, Married, Widowed, or Divorced (write word)_____

If married or widowed, husband of or wife of_____

(If husband, give wife's maiden name)

Birthplace_____City or Town———State or Country____

Mother's Maiden Name____Mother's Birthplace, State, or Country__

Father's Name_____Father's Birthplace, State, or Country__

Informant_____Address_____

Nearest Relative, Guardian, or Friend_____

Address_____ Telephone No._____

Referred by_____Referring Physician_____

HISTORY: *Present Illness:*_____

_____

_____

PAST HISTORY: Tuberculosis ____ Heart Disease__Cancer __Diabetes___

Mental Illness____Arthritis____Genitourinary Dis.___

PHYSICAL EXAMINATION ON ADMISSION by Attending Physician:

√ = normal findings

Head____Eyes____Ears____ Vision____ Hearing ____Teeth____

Heart_____   Lungs_____

Blood Pressure_____Pulse_____ Rhythm_____

Abdomen_____

Genitalia_____

Mental Status_____

Extremities_____

FUNCTIONAL CAPACITY: _____

LABORATORY: Urine   Blood examination   Hemoglobin___

Albumin_____   as indicated: Blood Sugar___

Sugar_____   Hematocrit____N.P.N___

DIAGNOSIS:

An abstract of the last hospital or nursing home admission with
diagnosis and summary of treatment should accompany this record.

Date_____   _____M.D.

FIG. 1

Admission record for chronic and convalescent nursing
homes.

first has to do with the patient's identity. The second section is for the patient's history; this includes the present illness and past history. To simplify the form, we have indicated in the past history those diseases that are most characteristic of the aging. The third section is for the physical examination; if the findings are normal, they need only be checked; if abnormal, they are described as they relate to that system of the body. Visual, circulatory, pulmonary, and neuromuscular systems are recorded, as are the patient's mental status and functional capacity. The fourth section is allotted to laboratory reports of urine analysis and blood examination. This information facilitates diagnosis, ensures adequate treatment, and outlines a program for the patient.

The nursing report (Figure 2) records an admission note on the patient's general condition, the presence of gross abnormal findings, and vital signs. The daily record then reports vital signs, medication, treatment, and general condition. If the patient becomes seriously ill, the temperature and vital signs are charted every four hours. A sheet is provided for both the doctor's orders and progress notes (Figure 3). Individual narcotic and sedative sheets are kept on patients receiving these drugs. Narcotics are checked for amounts ordered and administered. If the patient is admitted from a general hospital or other nursing home, an abstract of the record is required. As noted, the new Medicare Act requires the exchange of medical information between the hospital and the nursing home. Experience indicates that some general hospitals have in the past cooperated in transmitting this information; this interchange will undoubtedly improve under the new law. The medical records must be stored for 10 years.

| | | | | | | | | | | DAILY NOTES |
DATE	TEMP.	PULSE	RESP.	INTAKE	OUTPUT	BOWELS	DIET	HOUR	MEDICATIONS & TREATMENTS	(Including doctors' visits, all physical complaints)

NURSE'S REPORT

PATIENT'S NAME   ROOM NO.

FIG. 2

Nurse's report for nursing homes.

	DOCTOR'S ORDER SHEET AND PROGRESS NOTES	
	Patient's Name: _____	
	Diagnosis: _____	
	Doctor: _____	
DATE	ORDERS	PROGRESS NOTES

FIG. 3

Physician's order sheet and progress notes for the nursing home.

A good medical record assures that the patient has been carefully examined, that his physical condition has been appraised, and that proper treatment will be followed. Early recognition of disease and early treatment may prevent many complications in the elderly patient. Undiagnosed disease cannot be treated. The future planning of the patient's program in his new environment depends on his diagnosis and his functional capacities as they are evaluated by the physician in the record. The measure of effectiveness of any program is its acceptance and its use. Physicians and nurses will complete forms if they are applicable to the situation and are of assistance in their everyday work. Forms do not require the detail embodied in general hospital medical records because the services and requirements differ, but they should include the basic information.

The Nurse's Responsibility

It is necessary today to spread professional skills as widely as possible, while still providing good care. It is not sufficient for the registered nurse to see a few patients and leave many others to the care of the nurse's aides. While professional nursing skills must be available to every patient in the nursing home, there remains the question of how widely they can be spread. This will be a continuing and growing problem as the number of nursing homes increase. The 1962 U.S. Public Health survey showed that the majority of proprietary nursing homes providing skilled nursing care had no registered nurse on duty, and some 14 per cent had neither a registered nurse nor a licensed practical nurse—a fact that emphasizes both the shortage of qualified nurses and the need to improve nursing-home care.

One of the major functions of the nursing home is to provide skilled nursing care—not custodial care. The implementation in 1967 of the nursing-home section of the Medicare Act will undoubtedly speed this change of attitude, since the Act requires the employment of at least one registered nurse. Although many states already require this, many are lax in their enforcement and allow provisional nursing homes that provide sub-quality nursing service. Welfare agencies in many states contribute to this situation. The nursing supervisor must be a registered nurse who can perform those duties requiring special skills, as well as supervise and teach other attendants to carry out duties requiring less skill.

NURSE-PHYSICIAN RELATIONSHIP

The first responsibility of the registered nurse is to see that doctors' orders are carried out—that each patient receive his medicines and treatments as ordered. The registered nurse, of course, also administers medications. Furthermore, she should make rounds with the physician-in-charge and have regular conferences with him on each patient. As it is the responsibility of the nurse's aide to keep the supervisor informed, so the nursing supervisor must keep the doctor informed. Any change in the medical status of a patient should be called to the doctor's attention. Because of her daily association with the patient, the nursing supervisor sees the changes in his condition, and her observation can prove helpful to the physician.

It is the registered nurse's responsibility to call the physician in a medical emergency, a decision that should not be left to the nursing-home administrator or owner, any more than it would be to the administrator of a general hospital. This should be clearly understood by the nurse, the administrator, and the doctor. Since the physician is ultimately responsible for the quality of care in the nursing home, he must support the nurse's authority in medical matters.

TEAM NURSING

In team nursing the supervisor or charge nurse (who is a registered nurse) is the team leader. Registered nurses are trained to observe and recognize nursing needs. In a nursing home, it is possible to get to know and understand patients because of their longer stay. The supervisor should assess the needs of her patients with both the physician and with her aides and adjust nursing care to meet them. A patient may be blind, deaf, lame, confused, or frightened; alternatively, he may require only a feeling of security. Perhaps he requires help in hygiene or in daily activities; the emphasis should then be placed on these facets of his daily care. The professional nurse, who receives the reports from the licensed practical nurses and the nurse's aides, is in a position to recognize such needs and see that they are met. Some patients preparing to return home may need her special advice and assurance. She is called on to deal with many problems, from the prevention of bed sores and crippling contractions to those involving family relationships.

A registered nurse who acts as a nursing-home supervisor will find herself less concerned with the mechanics of the treatment ordered and the medicine to be dispensed than she will with the care of the whole patient.

Since care involves patients who may remain in the home for extended stays, she may need a considerable revision of viewpoint and be involved with matters that go beyond the basic necessity to see that the nursing reports and medical records are kept up to date. Such simple things as catering to an older person's whims in order to raise his morale assume unusual importance, as does the assignment of an aide to a particular patient with whom she strikes a sympathetic note.

The role of the team leader is especially demanding, generally involving the training of aides to care for the particular needs of patients in her absence. As the team leader, the registered nurse uses her judgment, skills, and knowledge to determine, not only the patient's needs, but the abilities of the workers as well. Which attendant can perform a particular service better than the others? Which of the workers on call can most nearly meet the patient's needs? The supervisor must determine that each aide who cares for a patient is aware of that individual's needs. The aide may require new instructions after several days off duty. The nursing team functions as a whole because the professional nurse plans the care for each patient on a round-the-clock basis and prepares a written plan for continuous care in her absence.

In team nursing, the team leader must assemble her staff daily to discuss the special needs of individual patients. These may involve range-of-motion problems or re-education in the activities of daily living, areas in which the nurse's aides may require instruction. Aides may serve as the eyes and ears of the supervisor, but never as her head. It is also the leader's responsibility to revise and change plans of care as conditions evolve.

The auxiliary personnel have the responsibility to

carry out their assignments, ask questions about their assignments, and familiarize themselves with the patient and his medical record. They may present their observations in conference, suggest alternative procedures, and seek advice on the best team approach to follow. The registered nurse gathers the pertinent information from their detailed reports of the patient's activities. Perhaps the family should visit the patient more often, or perhaps someone else should be assigned to this patient. Learning to conduct a conference can be difficult, but with experience the team leader and members learn to communicate and work together to do effective team nursing.

Many members of the nursing team are nurse's aides. It is important that the registered nurse make sure that the aides understand and learn to perform their duties through planned training and continuing education in those services and nursing procedures that require knowledge and skills beyond those possessed by the average person. This involves carrying out procedures in accordance with orders. The charge nurse must exercise care and judgment in assigning to the aides duties that are commensurate with their respective skills. To ensure safe practice, this personnel should be carefully screened and evaluated. The judgment of the professional nurse will determine the effectiveness of her teaching in the preparation of untrained people for assignment to nursing care. One can be certain that safe and comprehensive care will be given only when a sound training program has been organized.

First, the workers' abilities and the requirements of the job must be evaluated. This involves setting a pattern of duties and procedures, breaking them down to their simplest forms, and emphasizing key points. It requires the provision of necessary equipment and the gradual transfer of training from the classroom to the patient. Emphasis on basic duties is followed by consideration of the more complicated. By planning, teaching, and assignment of duties, the registered nurse and nursing attendants function as a team and can extend their skills efficiently.

Other Nursing-Home Personnel

As the standard of care is raised and the nursing homes become more medically oriented, the services of other professional persons will be required. This will probably be done on a part-time or consultation basis at first, both because there is a shortage of such personnel and because such services are expensive.

The services of a physical therapist, an occupational therapist, and a speech therapist are obviously invaluable for elderly patients. Although full-time employment of such a paramedical staff will necessarily be restricted to the largest homes, considerable benefit can accrue from part-time utilization of such services, both in teaching the nursing staff and in treating patients.

The role of the social worker in the nursing home has yet to be defined, despite the fact that social problems are frequently encountered in these patients. In New York City it was found that some patients could be returned to their homes or the homes of relatives through the efforts of a social service worker. This specialty will undoubtedly be used increasingly in the future.

A professionally trained dietitian should be employed by all nursing homes. In the smaller homes, because of costs, this may be necessary on a part-time basis. Elderly persons are often undernourished and frequently must eat a restricted diet because of diabetes, heart disease, or dental problems. This subject is discussed in detail in Chapter 5.

It should be remembered that all the professional people here considered are now employed at local general hospitals. It is hoped that, with the Medicare Act and as closer affiliations between hospitals and nursing homes are developed, the tremendous highly trained resources of the *hospital staff* may be utilized, *on a part-time or consultation basis by even the smaller nursing homes.*

3

Psychiatric Nursing of the Elderly Patient

―――・・・―――

The Evolving Role of the Nurse

During the past decade, the role of the nurse has changed greatly in many respects. Before World War II, she fulfilled two roles—the one for which she was trained and the other that reflected her own view of herself as a person attracted to a profession that cared for the sick. The emphasis in training was formerly directed to physical needs, ranging from care of a particular pathological condition to the more custodial aspects of environmental control. The development of medical specialization, however, has greatly altered the training and duties of nurses, as it has that of all affiliated professional groups.

The Changing Role of the Nurse

The ever-expanding increase in medical knowledge has brought about changes in the schedules of medical

students, interns, and residents. The expansion of medical services, accelerated by the rapid growth of the
population, has enforced more effective use of all available manpower; increasingly, some of the duties of
interns and residents have been delegated to nurses.
The field of anesthesiology exemplifies the emergence
of specialized nursing functions. To help her to meet
these added responsibilities, the nurse in training has
been therefore subjected more and more to an academic
curriculum to help her acquire a more basic knowledge
of medical subjects, but this has necessitated a reduction of time devoted to actual patient care. Social
trends, such as the shortened work week, have intensified these modifications in training and in work. The
prestige devolving on the nurse who performs duties
hitherto regarded as the functions of the physician has
influenced the directions in which the nursing profession has proceeded.

The public complains that the physician has become
a technician and no longer resembles the general medical practitioner. The image of the nurse has suffered
equally. Nurses are accused of paying more and more
attention to the technical aspects of patient care, with
a loss of the maternal qualities traditionally attributed
to them. There has been a marked diminution of the
attitude of regarding the patient as a human being
with fears and anxieties, the easing of which was a
primary obligation of both physician and nurse. The
expanded knowledge of pathology and a phenomenal
increase in the medical armamentarium have brought
about a change of focus; the patient is now regarded
as the carrier—or possessor—of a disease or a diseased
organ. Moreover, the availability of potent medication

has created a definite trend in the medical and nursing professions to disregard the psychological roles of the physician and nurse in enabling the patient to focus his potential to overcome the disease process.

The Evolving Role of the Physician

This change of attitude has other implications that relate to the development of personal prestige. The omnipotence attributed to the physician has diminished as the public has become increasingly educated in medical matters, as it has come to recognize the value of scientifically applied procedures in and out of medicine, and as it has become more familiar with the work of the medical and allied professions. The major casualty of these modifications has been the appreciation of the healing functions of the practitioner who enters into a close personal relationship with the person reduced by illness to dependency. Despite these changes, the average man becomes less sophisticated about medicine when he becomes sick. Often, however, he maintains the appearance of sophistication to some degree in order to bolster his own view of himself. There remains, however, the feeling of helplessness and the need for reassurance and comfort that can be given only by parental authority figures—that is, the physician and the nurse.

Evolution of the Doctor-Patient Relationship

An interesting aspect of the changing nature of the doctor-patient relationship is the fact that, corresponding to this decreasing interpersonal involvement, there has been a greater development of psychiatry. The psychiatrist appears to have assumed the role of the traditional physician to whom patient and family turn for personal support and help in the face of difficulty. Undoubtedly, one of the reasons for this development is the fact that the psychiatrist is regarded as a physician who is willing to listen to personal problems and to help the patient deal with his emotional reactions.

According to a number of surveys, the image of the physician has deteriorated markedly over the past two decades. The average person believes his own physician is different from the other members of the profession. Obviously, this separation is based on unconscious psychological factors. Similarly, while nurses may wish to regard themselves in part as physicians, scientists, or technicians, the public continues to view them in their traditional role. This observation would seem to be of a particular significance for nursing educators who aspire to train women for roles that eliminate completely their traditional attributes.

Education of the Modern Nurse

The alterations in the duties of the nurse over the past several decades have been designed mainly to permit her to fulfill her professional role. The performance of duties now regarded as housekeeping has been transferred to others. As a consequence, the nurse is increasingly regarded as an intelligent and educated person who should be encouraged to utilize her acquired skills, to develop her potential, and to assume increasing responsibility.

The responsibility for the performance of new functions and duties leads to a demand for a higher level of training and higher levels of professional education. If this new knowledge is to be taught during the basic training period, the duration of the educational process would necessarily be lengthened. Practical considerations that place limits on the length of training may well create a demand for specialization on the graduate level. Today, one of the major problems in the education of the student nurse in diploma training schools is to find adequate time for training in basic psychology as applied to patients.

The Nursing-Home Patient

Because this presentation is addressed primarily to nurses who are concerned with patients in chronic convalescent hospitals and in nursing homes, emphasis is laid on the psychological aspects of the nursing care of persons in the older age groups. Such homes are beginning to recognize the demand that they assume responsibility for persons suffering from chronic psychiatric illnesses, as well as for those with physical disabilities. There is a developing opinion that such persons, even if psychotically ill, need not be cared for in large, overcrowded psychiatric hospitals. This is especially true of the older patient who presents emotional problems of a nature not disturbing to others. Older people frequently present clinical pictures of emotional illness, even to a psychotic degree, although they require nursing care primarily for physical illness. Should not the older patient, whose primary need for care arises from emotional illness, also be tended in the same kind of institution? Many, if not the majority, of the older patients admitted to mental hospitals are individuals who, reacting partly to biological alterations and partly to environmental changes, can be comfortably managed in a setting that does not carry with it the stigma of a state mental hospital.

In a number of states, there is a developing movement to transfer many patients in the older age group from psychiatric hospitals to convalescent and chronic hospitals. So clear is the trend that one may assume that in the years ahead the chronic and convalescent hospital will assume a major responsibility for most elderly individuals presently diagnosed as mentally ill and requiring treatment in state institutions. One might even forecast that this will be true also for middle-aged persons who, unable to function as individuals within the community, require institutionalization. Evidence of these developments can be seen in the increasing numbers of emotionally ill patients now maintained outside the state mental hospital, either with the provision of foster care in the community or with nursing-home care.

Causes of Mental Changes in the Elderly Person

ORGANIC BRAIN DAMAGES

The general diagnostic approach to the illness of elderly persons, in the present as in the past, has been to regard them as suffering from organic brain damage and organic deterioration. The classic diagnostic symptoms of senility have included constrictions of interest, a tendency to irritability and liability of emotional reaction, a decline in personal care and hygiene, and an apparent indifference to the niceties of culture and speech. Lapses of memory, lack of initiative, and a preoccupation with the past have been attributed entirely to loss of function caused by organic brain damage. This view has seldom been challenged by physicians, including psychiatrists, largely because the life span of the average individual usually brought him to illness and death at an earlier age than today, when people live longer and require extended nursing care. As recently as two decades ago, it was always anticipated that a very large percentage of patients over the age of 65 admitted to mental hospitals would die within the first year. The evidence, therefore, seemed to support the view that psychiatric disturbance could be attributed only to organic brain disease.

There is a new realization, however, that the psychiatric illness of the elderly is the result of two basic processes: one organic, and less severe than formerly regarded; the other, psychological. With regard to organic brain changes, it is true that with increasing age there are changes in the brain. Individual brain cells deteriorate and die. With this occur certain signs in intellectual processes. On neurological examination, many changes are not of significance. They do not severely impair the normal motor activity of the individual except at a very late stage.

In his intellectual functioning, the elderly person shows increasing restriction of his areas of interest. He becomes less and less involved with the world around him and more and more concerned with himself and his immediate environment. These changes arise, not so much because of brain damage or deterioration as because the environment ceases to attract or stimulate him. He lives increasingly in an environment of younger people who have interests different from his. As he and his contemporaries become less mobile in a world that is increasingly mobile, his contacts with persons of his own age and interests gradually diminish. With less stimulation from the wider environment, his interests and energies become focused on his immediate surroundings—and on himself. He may feel neglected, unimportant, and useless. As his resentment smolders, he can be quickly annoyed. He may eventually focus his attention entirely on himself and on his memories of a past that is pleasant to recall. He becomes indifferent to those he feels are indifferent to him; consequently, he becomes indifferent to such rules for conforming to social behavior as attention to personal attire and personal hygiene.

PSYCHOLOGICAL STRESS

There is little doubt that many of the behavioral symptoms that appear in elderly persons can be attributed more to psychological causes than to organic brain disease. Even diminished perception of the physical surroundings appears to arise from loss of interest rather than from impairment of the perceptual apparatus.

It is too seldom recognized that many elderly persons develop neurotic conditions, anxiety states, depressive reactions, and even phobic reactions. The psychological process of aging may commence well before the age of 65. As a man approaches the age of 60, he has in general reached the peak of his standard of living. Future advancement, vocational or financial, is likely to be negligible. Ahead looms nothing but retirement and the prospect of a lower income, a lower standard of living, and perhaps dependence on others. The prospect of economic deprivation reinforces the effects of frustrated ambition. Anxiety gradually arises. Decreased levels of performance in several areas of life augment this anxiety. Minor illnesses raise the specter of serious incapacitating conditions and even death.

Depressive reactions become more frequent, but usually not to such a degree as to be clinically obvious. Rather, they may be evidenced by loss of initiative, by increased withdrawal, and sometimes by increased use of alcohol. In their early stages, these emotional reactions may not be evident even to the individual. Elderly persons may not voice their concerns because their psychological defenses operate to keep their fears out of their consciousness. However, one who is skilled, knowledgeable, and sensitive may pick up clues to these concerns while engaging the individual in conversation.

With actual retirement, the picture may immediately become very clear. Not infrequently, however, the more severe reactions are delayed for a time because the individual has for so long deluded himself about his happy state when he no longer needs to work. He anticipates a freedom to do what he likes when he likes. Within a year or less, the "bloom is off the rose." Many hours once occupied by vocational activities must now be filled. Moreover, he lacks the companionship of those with whom he worked, while decreased economic circumstances severely limit the ambitions he entertained regarding the use of his leisure. The monotony of the day stretches out endlessly before him.

Senescence, the period of normal aging, thus becomes

a time of psychological stress. Some elderly persons develop neurotic symptoms around instinctual drives generally regarded as the perogatives of the young. The sexual drive may often diminish and disappear, at least in direct expression; however, it may persist in older people and become a serious source of difficulty. Normal sexual activity may be blocked for a variety of reasons and may be evidenced in fondling or pinching those who are not the natural objects of the individual's sexual relationship. Alternatively, severe guilt reactions may be occasioned by fantasies that do not physically involve others. Conversion reactions may occur—that is, the individual develops an impairment of function in an area of the body under the control of the voluntary nervous system, such as the muscles or limbs. As in the younger person, such symptoms are the results of the psychological defenses the individual adopts to protect himself from his own unacceptable drives.

Under sufficient stress, an individual of any age may regress psychologically. In the elderly, regression to levels of psychological and social adjustment typical of early childhood is very frequent because the environment tends to enhance any tendency to withdrawal and to fantasy. When there are also internal drives that are unacceptable to the superego (or conscience), the pressures toward regression may become irresistible, with a return to a level of infantile adjustment. Conflicts of an adult nature are thus avoided; at the same time, emotional support and reassurance may be forthcoming from those about him.

One aspect of the life patterns of the elderly is the limitation of available or potential emotional support. The child automatically turns to a parent for reassurance; the young adult has recourse to older adults; the older adult can turn at least to friends of his own age. Few individuals turn to others of younger age and of less experience. The elderly person is in a different situation; there are few individuals of his own or greater age to whom he can turn. Handicapped by a reduced circle of acquaintances and friends and shut off from former colleagues at work, the elderly person is relatively isolated. He is obliged to seek emotional support from younger individuals—a position not regarded as reassuring at any age and in fact destructive of self-esteem and self-respect. It is in this situation that the physician and the nurse, who psychologically carry the images and authority of parents, can be particularly helpful and effective because the elderly person is able to relate to them emotionally and can accept their instructions and guidance without a loss of self-respect.

The problem of the relative importance of organic brain disease and psychological stress in the causation of symptoms is perhaps best illustrated in the case of a moderately severe depression in the elderly. Many older persons suffer from this disorder. They exhibit the typical signs: loss of appetite and initiative, with changes in food patterns and increasing immobility. There is insomnia, with reduced hours of sleep and early waking; indifference to personal attire; and slovenliness. These symptoms of depression may be seen in individuals at all ages after puberty. When seen in the person over 65, they are almost automatically diagnosed as irreversible senile brain deterioration because symptoms of depression in the elderly have been regarded as the classic signs of brain organicity. It is probable that, of the large number of diagnosed senile cases in mental hospitals, a considerable proportion are primarily cases of affective disorders that would respond to a few electroshock treatments. Because of physical and legal risks, these patients never have the opportunity to receive the treatment that might remove the symptoms and restore them to more normal function.

Psychiatric Role of the Nurse

In the more specialized programs of psychiatric nursing education, emphasis is placed on the importance of the nurse's working with the patient as an individual person, forming a relationship with him, and identifying his psychological problems. This is, in part, a return to the effective use of the nurse in her traditional role. The modern trend toward nurses who are mechanically perfect technicians has thus given rise to a reactionary trend. The psychiatric nurse in a very small number of psychiatric nurse training programs is being educated to be relatively—if not completely—disinterested in all the techniques involving physical nursing care and to be interested mainly in the beneficial effects of the nurse-patient relationship.

In most general nursing education programs, the emphasis on physical care is compensated for by a psychiatric affiliation for three months, during which the student nurse gains psychological insights through her work with psychiatric patients. It is interesting to note how seldom these student nurses are capable of talking to patients as people. They ask for instructions as to how they should talk to them; they manifest obvious embarrassment when called upon to be natural in their relationships with them. Having learned to relate to patients as the possessors of pathological organs and as the objects on which to perform technical procedures, they now require instruction in what was once the nurse's most important function.

Ideally, therefore, the nurse working with psychologically ill persons, with or without secondary emotional reactions, must have the skills to meet both physical and psychological needs. It is as dangerous for the nurse to lose sight of the physical needs of the emotionally ill under her care as it is to treat the individual only as a mechanical robot. The modern concept of psychiatry is to regard the psyche and the soma as aspects of a single, indivisible entity that may be viewed from two aspects, the somatic and the psychological, just as one may view a table from different angles; the front and side differ in aspect, but are only separate views of a single entity.

COMMUNICATION BETWEEN NURSE AND PATIENT

Similarly, when one regards a person, one may see only a superficial aspect, the skin. Nevertheless, beneath it lie unseen the organs that comprise the functioning entity. Looking at the individual from the psychological vantage point, one may see only the conscious part of his psyche; under the surface lie the unconscious structures that are essential to his psychological functioning. It is well to remember this because in a relationship between two people, especially in a therapeutic one, a great deal of communication occurs on the unconscious level. With respect to the nurse, this communication operates at the level of a mother-child relationship. Some nurses have no mothering characteristics and willingly dispense with them because they reject any effectiveness not based on intellectual ability or skill. The parallel with the father-child relationship of the physician-patient is clear.

With regard to psychiatric diagnosis, the definition of mental or emotional illness may commence with observations of a person's behavior as it differs from that of an individual in the same social, educational, and vocational position. Alternatively, the changes in a person's behavior may be of such proportions that he is obviously different from the original person. Thus, the diagnosis of mental illness is often based on the observations of others, the precise diagnostic category depending on the varieties of behavioral pictures.

The individual, while rarely thinking of himself initially as a psychiatric patient, often recognizes that he differs from his previous self. He wants help from others —even though at times his reactions appear to deny the validity of this need. Most individuals suffering from psychiatric disorders have genuine difficulty in communicating with others. The aim of the psychotherapist is to establish communication, primarily on verbal level. Psychiatrists recognize the possibility even more communication may occur on the nonverbal level—through gestures, muscular reactions and movements, and tone of voice, for example. Often of greatest importance in determining the success or failure of establishing communication is the manner in which the therapist reacts to the antagonism, anger, or rejection expressed by the patient. The therapist who is not experienced, knowledgeable, and skilled may react with negative emotions, so demonstrating to the patient that he does not understand the nature of the relationship. This is comparable to the hostile reactions that some patients exhibit to their physicians after surgery.

Fears and anxieties temporarily overwhelm other aspects of a patient's personality to throw him into a state of emotional instability that leads him to the nearest person for his distress. The same considerations apply in all cases of illness, whether the patient be in a general hospital, a psychiatric facility, or a chronic and convalescent hospital. The physician and the nurse must learn to view such behavior objectively and must not react personally to abuse.

In order to be able to do this in a professional manner, the nurse, like the doctor, must learn about the motivations of such behavior. Often careful thought will create an understanding of the stresses to which the person is exposed; with this knowledge, forebearance and tolerance become easier.

Persons responsible for the care of the sick should also be familiar with the area of self-recognition. They must understand their customary ways of reacting to anger, resentment, and abuse. They must learn how one becomes emotionally involved with a patient, sometimes developing positive or negative feelings without reason. They must learn why one sometimes spends a great deal more time with some patients and a minimum with others, even when the latter should be receiving the most attention. Even the average healthy mother who loves her child will sometimes feel that she cannot bear with him much longer and that she would be happier if he were elsewhere. Such emotional reactions are of short duration and are often limited by intellectual recognition of the child's dependency. Similiar situations arise frequently with patients with psychiatric problems. It is much easier to react "naturally" —that is, as if the patient were a normal person with full intellectual abilities and complete responsibility. This is an emotional reaction. On the other hand, one can isolate one's emotions completely and regard the patient abstractly, understanding in a rational manner that he is emotionally disturbed and that one must perform one's duties as a technician without becoming involved. This is the purely intellectual approach. With knowledge and training, it is not too difficult to acquire.

The ideal involves a more difficult approach. One must learn that the reactions of the patient are not directed to the nurse as an individual unless, of course, she provokes them. These reactions are to be recognized as manifestations of the patient's difficulties with himself and his environment. They represent methods by which the patient is coping with inner distress. At the same time, the patient needs someone with whom to form a relationship, someone who can accept the temporary anger and still continue to be warm and friendly and understanding. With patients in the older age group, this is especially true because their emotional reactions tend to be sudden and severe but of short duration, not unlike those of the young child. This is especially true when the clinical condition is one of regression to earlier childhood patterns—the "second childhood" of literature.

PHYSICAL CONTACT

One of the differences between the psychotherapy of younger persons and the care of the older individual lies in the philosophy about physical contact. In the former, there is usually no physical contact between patient and doctor. With the therapy of frankly psychotic persons, the patient may need and benefit from some physical contact. With the elderly person, physical care may be very important because it represents contact with real persons, for many of them have had loss of contact with people they knew and loved. Physical contact, such as the arm around the shoulder, is often emotionally a very supportive measure for those individuals who are as depressed as many elderly patients are. At any age, "crying on the shoulder" of another who is seemingly strong and capable of protecting, just as the hurt child runs to its mother, is a usual manifestation of need for support. With such elderly patients, demonstrations of this nature have emotionally charged symbolic meanings and are powerful aids in giving reassurance.

VERBAL CONTACT

Patients in nursing homes are by definition in need of long-term care. The relationship of nurse and patient must be seen as long-term; the nurse, therefore, may apply many techniques to encourage the patient to become involved. One such method involves merely sitting with the patient, passing an occasional comment, asking an appropriate question, and above all entering into conversation on topics of interest to the patient. Often when one learns the patient's past interests, occupation, and avocational pursuits, one may begin to establish a relationship by having the patient discuss or describe these facets of his life. Because they are dependent, patients may respond to repeated little services. They can be coaxed and their mood changed by distracting attention from unpleasant to pleasant topics, as with children.

It must never be obvious, however, that they are being treated like children. They must be made to feel that they remain individuals who are respected by those on whom they are dependent. This is not quickly or easily accomplished.

It is not necessary to engage them in incessant conversation. The model is the home setting, where members of the family pursue their varied interests and activities individually; when the mood prevails or the occasion arises, conversation ensues about some pertinent topic or point of information. With the elderly, the number of advances must be greater in order repeatedly to stimulate the interest of the patient and to condition him to the fact that the nurse is an integral part of his environment. Marked changes can be effected in transforming an apparently apathetic senile individual into a reasonably alert and responsive person by the persistence and perseverance of the nursing staff. Not least important is establishing the patient's independence by his ability to move about.

The latter improvement is an example of the importance of the combination of emotional support and of physical contact and physical care—a point that cannot be overemphasized. The need for physical touch and support in helping an individual overcome his fears in order to restore his mobility is very well recognized in the aftermath of acute illnesses. With the regressed patient, the procedures require even more frequent and persistent application. He requires a type of reconditioning akin to that of the early years when he first learned to walk.

If the nurse-patient relationship is so important, the question may be raised as to the desirability of changing assignments of the nursing staff. Should the same nurse remain always with the same patients? Two considerations enter the picture—one theoretical and psychological, the other a practical one.

Theoretically it is desirable to keep the same nurse with the same patient as the latter establishes a relationship of importance to him. Change of assignments without further contact may be interpreted in a variety of ways, all undesirable in their effects. The degree of commitment of the individual nurse to her patients is important. On the other hand, staffing patterns may necessitate a rotational system. On occasion, it is necessary to relieve a nurse who is carrying a particularly stressful assignment. Even when changes are necessary, ideally, the relationship should be maintained by arranging to have the nurse visit those patients with whom she has established important interactions.

Although great stress is laid on the need for a richness of human contact for these old persons, this does not imply that they should never be left alone. For many, short periods of being alone may be important. There is a world of difference between being lonely and being alone. The latter usually implies a temporary isolation from others, sometimes without choice, but often by decision of the individual himself. Some people wish to be left alone for such periods.

Loneliness, on the other hand, is an emotional state, a distressing emotion implying loss or absence of persons to whom one can relate in a human way. Many, if not the majority, of elderly persons entering institutions know this feeling. It often lies at the root of the psychiatric disorders of old age. There is opportunity for the exercise of great skill in nursing these patients so that the aching void can be filled, at least in part. This is one of the prime objectives of good psychiatric nursing, expressed in technical language as "establishing a meaningful relationship with the patient."

Characteristics of Older Patients

THE PSYCHIATRIC DIAGNOSTIC LABEL

One type of problem arising in nursing homes is that occasioned by the admission of a patient with a psychiatric diagnosis and who has been transferred from a state or private psychiatric hospital. The psychiatrically uneducated and inexperienced nurse entertains many anxieties and fears because her image of the psychiatrically ill patient is one of potential violence. In fact, the majority of such patients tend to be docile. The old image of the mental patient as a violent one has a long tradition originating in the days when only the very disturbed were apprehended and incarcerated. Another factor influencing this image is the general recognition of the fact that many capital crimes are obviously the acts of mentally ill persons. Nevertheless, except for irrascibility and its consequences, most psychiatric patients demonstrate no trend toward physical abuse of others; they are neither troublesome nor difficult.

Thus, when patients are transferred to nursing homes from state mental hospitals "on trial visit," the significance of the phrase should be understood. The procedure is largely administrative. A patient on "trial visit" status can be readmitted to the state hospital without the formalities that attend a new admission. If for any reason the patient is unsuited to the nursing home, his return to the hospital is easily arranged. The term "on trial visit" therefore does not imply an expectation on the part of the psychiatrist that the patient will become difficult or impossible to manage—much less that he will be destructive. Many elderly patients in mental hospitals are quiet and well-behaved and should not be there; they belong in nursing homes.

These patients do exhibit psychiatric symptoms. They may have obvious delusional beliefs—the old woman who is afraid that there is a man under her bed or the man who ritualistically and constantly walks in some particular pattern, for example, in a circle. It is useless to try to talk them out of such symptoms by trying to convince them of the falseness of the belief or the uselessness of the ritual. The best approach is to engage them in other activities. When their interest is aroused, they are less preoccupied with their symptoms. Again, it may be pointed out that knowledge of the patient's past or present interests offers one of the best avenues for developing such a program.

With regard to the woman who believes there is a man in her room, one should not in any way reinforce her delusional belief by, for example, saying that the man will be taken out. Although the lady does not actually see this imaginary man, he symbolizes her unconscious wishes and conflicts. Therefore, any attempt to convince her that he is nonexistent can only lead to disagreement. She needs that man—she has probably had him for a long time! It is more important to recognize the fact that the symptom represents an unconscious wish that is unacceptable to her conscience. Therefore, the approach should be to distract her from her preoccupation by engaging her in conversation about her past, her familial experiences, her successes and her disappointments or, at a later stage, her anxieties about herself.

DISORIENTATION

A particular problem with older persons is the disorientation that occurs in the dark. Many elderly persons become extremely anxious and fearful, even delusional and hallucinated, when they are moved from their familiar home environment to that of a hospital or nursing home. These disturbances are further intensified by turning off the light at night. This is because all persons establish their security vis-à-vis their physical environment by observing it and orienting themselves in that particular place. Anxious individuals are more anxious in new surroundings than are emotionally secure persons. From birth, every individual perceives his immediate environment and pictures everything in relation to himself. With familiarity, one comes to accept one's surroundings without conscious awareness.

With old age and with the psychological restriction of interest, one's emotional security becomes bounded also by an increasing restriction in one's physical environment. With the emotional problems attendant on advancing years, feelings of security sometimes become associated with a single room. Thus, an older person living alone will frequently restrict his or her life to only one room in the house, eating, living, and sleeping there.

Removal to new surroundings disrupts the life pattern of the already anxious individual whose capacity to learn and to manipulate ideas and concepts is grossly impaired. Darkness, therefore, produces a sense of loss of position in space. It is akin to the fears of the very

young child afraid of the dark in which he visualizes—
and hallucinates—all kinds of fearful beings. Like the
child, the older person is more secure sleeping in a
lighted room. For the same reason, the sleeping quarters of such persons should not be changed except for
the most pressing considerations.

Conclusions

In reviewing the developments in the field of nursing
over the past quarter century and current trends, one
sees major changes in both the function and the image
of the nurse. Her nonprofessional duties—that is, duties
not immediately related to the care of the patient—
have been transferred to others. This has freed much
of her time and energy, created in her a greater awareness of her professional role, and opened the door to
her undertaking of some duties previously performed
by physicians.

These changes were accompanied by education in
greater depth, the development of specialization, and
the focusing of attention on the pathological component
of the patient and techniques designed to hasten a
cure. Diminished awareness of the psychological and
emotional reactions of the patient as a person paralleled
this emphasis on the technical aspects of patient care.

In the 1960s, a number of trends forecast major
changes, and some previous trends have been reversed.
The emotional needs of the patient are being increasingly recognized, and psychiatric nursing has been introduced into the educational programs. This has occasionally proceeded to the development of postgraduate psy-

chiatric nursing programs with a graduate degree. As standards rise, the unfulfilled demand for more specialized instructors has intensified. At the same time, the need for trained nurses at the previous level of nursing practice has increased and has led to the acceptance of the licensed practical nurse as a person trained and qualified to perform practically all the duties that were assigned to the average registered nurse thirty or more years ago.

However, another trend is becoming evident. The diploma or hospital nursing schools are encountering problems in recruitment, in hiring trained instructors, and in financial matters. Many have already closed, and it is obvious that many others will follow their example in the near future. Since the demand for trained nurses will grow, the shortened educational program for the licensed practical nurse appears to be the best method of meeting this urgent need. The future pattern may well embrace the highly trained college nurse who will assume administrative and instructional duties, the registered nurse who will perform specialized patient-care functions, and the licensed practical nurse who will attend to immediate personal nursing needs. All classes of nurses, however, will be more adequately trained to be aware of the emotional needs of the patient, without regard to his particular disease. The patient will be treated as the most important person—as a human being.

4

The Nurse–Patient Relationship

———◆•◆———

THE NURSE caring for patients must learn to communicate and to relate herself to her charges. This is a new experience, one for which she must develop new attitudes. In everyday life, one is accustomed to communicating with healthy persons who are able to care for their own wants. In our social lives we can readily handle these contacts and relationships. We encourage those that we enjoy and that give mutual satisfaction and avoid those that do not. However, in interaction with patients, nurses cannot—if they are to give each sick person his due—use the technique of avoidance. When this widely used technique is employed, the quality of nursing care deteriorates, and the individuals on whom it is practiced are deprived of some of their primary rights and needs: the need to love and be loved, the need for acceptance, the need to preserve one's intrinsic worth and dignity, and the need for a feeling of personal worth.

The Nurse's Attitude

The fostering of a good nurse–patient relationship is a two-way process. Since one of the elements in the development of this relationship is the nurse, she must know herself before she can hope to make progress in understanding others. She must be able to recognize her own feelings and emotional reactions to patient behavior and learn to deal with these feelings so that they will not interfere with good patient care. A nurse is certain to have both positive and negative reactions to patients, which is the normal response of all human beings to each other. She needs to recognize the negative feelings for what they are so that they will not block her ability to see things from the patient's point of view.

She must also be sensitive to the reaction that she produces in others. It is just as important to assess this quality in terms of positive, meaningful reactions as in negative ones. Such self-awareness enables the nurse to sharpen and improve the qualities that invoke positive responses and facilitates her discovery in herself of those characteristics that require change or modification. The nurse may well be more important to her patients as an individual person than in her role as a technician.

How does one go about developing the self-awareness that creates an honest concept of oneself as a professional? A nurse who not only gives direct care, but also supervises the work of auxiliary personnel and who helps these people to develop their potential can check inappropriate reactions, especially when they recur. She can examine what preceded, what caused, and what succeeded an incident and seek for clues. This can be done in a number of ways: by reporting the incident in writing, by discussing it with an objective person, or by taking it up in group discussion. She can review what she knows about personality development and the defense mechanisms everyone uses to maintain equilibrium. She can examine interpersonal situations, on the job and off the job, and through contemplation and perhaps the guidance of others achieve an understanding of the factors that facilitate or hinder personal relationships. She must keep an open mind about her own behavior and the behavior of others, trying frankly and consciously to assess her own behavior, feelings, attitudes, and responses to various problems and situations.

The feeling of anger—a negative feeling to which all human beings are prone—deserves some attention. As "angels of mercy," nurses are apt to deny anger, which has many causes. Only the individual can know the reasons for his own anger: interference with a desired goal, personal or group injustice, the patients' tendency to refuse to help themselves and to make unreasonable demands, and being ignored. Since she has been taught to believe that nurses do not show anger toward patients, she feels guilty and avoids her charges when she fails them in this respect. In certain circumstances, however, anger may have some positive values: it may impel the individuals to improve an unsatisfactory situation. Such deliberate and therapeutic use, of course, demands study and control. Although it is true that nonverbal behavior—the way one looks, the tone of voice, and the type of touch—express both positive and negative feelings in a way that gets through to patients, the verbal expression of anger must be used with care, if at all. Change is the responsibility of the nurse, not the patient. No matter what the cause, the nurse should learn to express anger in ways that are not displayed toward the patient. She must accept and profit by the concept that all behavior is meaningful. Thus, no matter what the behavior that aroused the anger, the nurse should look within herself for the cause rather than show anger toward the patient, since his behavior, too, has a meaning. She must come to realize that anger is not only overtly aggressive, but can be expressed in subtle ways of avoidance: for instance, in forgetting food preferences, in delay in answering a call bell, and in a dozen other ways that come readily to mind.

A nurse's attitudes and reactions to a patient may be influenced by any or all of the following:

1. A nurse may expect of herself more than is humanly possible; therefore, in order to live with herself, she defensively says that patient Doe is creating problem.
2. There are diseases and conditions for which there is no cure; the patient may even resist attempts to help. This is most frustrating to the nurse.
3. There may be things about a patient—odors, morals, manners, and emotional outbursts, for example—that conflict with the nurse's sense of propriety to create a climate of nonacceptance.
4. The "Nightingale" veneer wears thin as the day goes on, and to her surprise the nurse finds herself snapping. The understanding nurse recognizes that the cause is her own fatique. The less sophisticated says, "Mr. X is impossible," and claims that "he would try the patience of a saint."

5. Although it is normal to wish to be liked by others, this desire can become a problem and the patient whom the nurse tries to please can become a burden. Our tendency to "keep smiling" and "to grin and bear it" becomes a burden. This compulsion builds up tensions within the nurse and within the patient who is expected to conform to this tradition. His frequent failure to conform subtly creates a feeling of disappointment.

What does the nurse do about her feelings concerning the patient who prefers to die now instead of waiting patiently? How does she handle the patient who defies all dietary instructions? How does she treat the martyr who resists medication or the patient who demands medication constantly? How does she deal with the differing reactions to pain by patients from different cultural backgrounds?

The Patient's Attitude

The patient in the hospital, cut off from his friends and his former world is lonely. New routines and uncertainties in a strange new home increase his fears. Added to this are often suffering and pain to deepen his despair. The patient seeks understanding and reassurance and looks to the nurse to share with him these experiences of loneliness. He turns to her for her human understanding as well as her nursing skills.

If the nurse is to care for him properly, she must know his point of view. What does he know about being ill, about the hospital world and the people in it?

e himself as a very sick person,
he has never known. He says to
them? I don't know anything
ow is that it will cost me a lot of
on these people to make me well."
is: "Can I trust these people?" The
re can be very disturbing to the pa-
helped to orient himself every step of
urse must remember that she is accus-
strange place; in a sense it is her home
ws every turn in the corridor and every
loor.

Patient "Categories"

Individuals do not like to be put in categories. Despite this, there will be on the fringe of each nurse's
consciousness categories into which she places her patients. It is far easier to categorize than it is to attempt
to understand the behavior that causes this categori-
zation.

Gertrude Ujhely, in her book *The Nurse and Her
Problem Patients,* lists some thirteen categories, including problem families. She makes no attempt to cover
them all. We, too, can select a few that are particularly
applicable to nursing-home situations. These summaries
of specific categories consider (1) what each type of
patient does, (2) the possible explanation for his behavior, and (3) the obligation each situation places on
the nurse involved. Here, in summary, are the categories
that may apply to the nursing-home situation.

THE UNCOOPERATIVE PATIENT

This type of patient sets up a barrier to and refuses all help, threatens the nurse's image of herself as a healer, and tends to destroy her picture of herself as a person of authority. This well may stem from his fear of accepting the reality of his illness or from lack of trust in the nurse's competence. All this imposes on the nurse the obligation to distinguish between the feeling that the patient's lack of cooperation is disturbing because he ignores her and the reality that it should be disturbing because it harms him. Once she accepts this viewpoint, she becomes objective and comes to appreciate the validity of the patient's viewpoint. This, in turn, frees her to help the patient to express himself as a step to discovering the basis of his resistance. Generally, direct questioning will fail to reveal this basis; attentive and analytic listening, however, may reveal clues to his reaction.

THE PATIENT WHO BECOMES PERSONAL

Many nurses are made uncomfortable by patients who become personal. Hildegarde Peplau, in her article "Talking with Patients," explains the reasons for not making a friend of a patient. If one stops to define a friend as a person one loves, with whom one shares confidences and experiences, it is obvious that few patients can become this close. One can be *friendly* without becoming a friend. The necessary nurse-patient relationship makes it impossible for a nurse to establish real friendships with the hundreds of patients for whom she cares. This type of patient may attempt to derive from the relationship more than the circumstances warrant, may exhibit a curiosity about the nurse's personal life, and may be overtly sexual or overtly motherly in his or her approach.

Such behavior has several possible explanations. It may be an attempt to disguise inadequacy; thus, a response to sexual suggestion or to mothering may reassure the patient as to his continuing ability in these areas. Alternatively, it may be the only pattern an individual has in relating to others. Then, too, the patient may feel that establishing a personal relationship will assure more favors. Finally, a man may be feeling helpless and in need of mothering. Since grown men are not supposed to need such consolation, this is converted to amorousness, which may be more acceptable in adults.

The nurse's reaction to such approaches must sooner or later involve a definition of the limits of the relationship. While we speak glibly of meeting a patient's needs, we must remember that one person cannot satisfy all demands and that the real need may be hidden and never expressed. Further, the nurse is entitled to safeguard her private life and should be firm in her refusal to give out personal information while simultaneously and tactfully developing a quiet relationship focused on the patient. Finally, without accepting or brusquely rejecting seductive advances, she can tactfully probe to discover their meaning and significance in the individual case.

THE NEGATIVE PROGNOSIS AND THE DYING PATIENT

This patient involves the nurse in psychological difficulties because he reminds her that she, too, is mortal; because he may cause her to feel that her healing ministry is futile; and, finally, because he may cause her to relive a personal grief or tragedy. Unlike the patient in other difficult situations, he does not will this and has no control over it; it is simply the product of a deteriorating state of body and mind. In this situation the nurse can do little more than attend meticulously to the patient's needs after clarifying her own feelings and perhaps learning to relegate them to the background. This she can do only by exploring her own feelings about death and rationalizing her attitude toward the dying patient in terms of refusing to attribute the natural fear we all share to her patient's condition. An acquaintance with the various ethnic, religious, and cultural attitudes toward death may prove very helpful in this respect.

THE OVERLY DEPENDENT PATIENT

The patient in this category, especially if allowed to become completely dependent, clings like a barnacle. He defeats the nurse's efforts to bring him to that evolving state of dependence, interdependence, and independence through which patients should proceed in a recovery process. This situation may prove very irritating to a nurse who herself has something of a dependent nature. Quite naturally, her reaction may be one of frustration that inevitably leads her to employ a technique of avoidance. The adult patient may be helpless in this situation; factors that he can normally control may now overwhelm him; and personal problems may prove beyond his capacity to handle during illness. Since his illness requires all his energy, he may now be overwhelmed by unfulfilled childhood needs, an awareness of which he was previously able to suppress. Any number of such factors may combine to place him in a situation of serious psychological distress.

In this situation, the nurse must come to grips with her own feelings about dependency, perhaps analyzing her upbringing and the role that dependency and self-sufficiency played therein. She should realize that she and her patient are two different people and should not impose on the patient her expectations of herself. Without pushing herself into the foreground, she makes herself available for reasonable demands from the patient's point of view. Thus, she can hope to support the patient until he gathers enough strength to move ahead independently. If this approach fails, she can always bring his behavior to the attention of the psychiatric service.

THE PATIENT WHO IS COMPLAINING AND DEMANDING

This type of patient may call for pain relievers periodically and may raise commotions that disturb other patients and set off chain reactions of dissatisfaction. He invariably attempts to manipulate the nurses to gain attention. The mainsprings of his action are not far to seek. It may be that the chronic nature of his disease changes his feelings of worth. His visitors grow fewer as the length of his stay in the home is extended. He becomes bored by his surroundings. He begins to understand that his illness is of little interest to others and thus begins to lose his sense of identity and importance.

The nurse's role in this situation is clear. She must hold the scales equal among her patients and not be goaded into misuse of her authority in response to irritation. This requires her to guard against redirecting other hostilities toward her patient and to continue to be concerned with his rights. There must be no power struggle between nurse and patient. She can achieve a stable situation if she will carefully consider the stress of long-term illness, reduce her own anxieties in order to keep those of her patient at a minimum, and use every possible nursing procedure to make her patient comfortable and bolster his sense of importance.

THE INCONTINENT PATIENT

No one with an active dislike of incontinence should be assigned to patient care. Incontinence is much more unpleasant in an adult than in an infant. Many nurses cannot contemplate bowel movements in an elderly person with equanimity; this is a regression to childhood. A nurse can change a child's diaper in the middle of preparing dinner, but find it difficult or impossible to perform the same service for an elderly invalid. It is difficult to rationalize the difference in attitude toward this problem in invalid adults and in infants. One can only recognize its existence and hope to revise it by an appreciation of the invalid's problems. The fact that incontinence creates problems of uncleanliness, including odor, that it creates laundry problems, and that it contributes to skin breakdown should be considered in relation to the possible causes. It may well be attributed to lack of patience or time on part of personnel for toilet training. The incontinence may be caused by lack of muscle tone or other organic factors. It may be that the patient, fearing bed sores, may thus hope to attract greater attention to the condition of his skin. Finally, psychological factors may play a part. The patient may be completely disoriented or may have regressed to a point of requiring to be cared for once more as an infant.

The nurse can cope with this situation in a variety

of ways. Primarily, she can give enough attention to obviate accidents. She can try to understand that her reactions to excreta are cultural rather than factual. She can try to revise her difference in attitude toward babies and elderly persons. She can endeavor to understand that to help with bedpans is a natural part of her task and that this does not detract from her dignity as a nurse. Above all, she must avoid scolding her patient and help him to retain a sense of dignity. She must help him in his bewilderment and understand that he may be very upset and distressed by the position in which his incompetence places him.

PATIENTS OF ADVANCED AGE

There is a wide gulf, involving more than a difference in years, between young personnel and extremely aged patients. In addition to presenting the problems of incontinence already discussed, they may turn night into day, show distrust toward everyone with whom they come into contact, may use insulting language to personnel and relatives, and may indulge in self-pity to an unrealistic degree. Occasionally, they harbor paranoid ideas which they project upon other patients in their immediate enviroment.

The conduct of these patients is usually based on recognizable reactions. As with all institutionalized patients, they may find it difficult to reconcile themselves to physical dependence, which is occasionally compounded by serious financial problems. They are convinced that their children no longer need or want them, partly because there is no one to care for them in an economy where almost everyone works. They may be so confused that no explanation seems to make sense to them. This feeling may be compounded by a conviction that hospitals are places to which people are relegated to die.

In this situation, the nurse's duty involves an obligation to assess the frustrations of deceleration and senescence and to consider how a limited income and terror of large hospital bills may affect the patient. Each service may seem to represent another item added to the bill. The nurse should attempt to ease the strangeness of an environment that increases the patient's natural confusion by changing things as little as possible and planning routines to meet the patient's desires when this is feasible. She must be prepared to answer the same questions repeatedly and anticipate that confusion may lead to panic and ideas of persecution. Her task will be facilitated if she will undertake to reorient the patient daily, and if she will allow him to make as many of his own decisions as are consistent with safety.

PROBLEM FAMILIES

The nursing home presents many problems that involve an understanding of family situations. The following guidelines will aid in assessing the effects of the family on the patient. In general, families may intrude at inopportune times and often may upset the patient with their emotionalism. In the presence of the patient, they may ask embarrassing questions that should be discussed privately with the physician. They may add to the difficulty of the nurse's task by demanding services to which they are not entitled. They may subtly suggest that the patient is being neglected and may reinforce this attitude by offering bribes to ensure special attention to the patient. At the other extreme, they may fail to visit the patient, even at long intervals.

Such family motivations may be understood in the context of guilt. This may be caused by a feeling that, by putting the patient in a nursing home, they have violated a cultural tradition that they should care for the aged at home. The sense of guilt may be exacerbated by recollections of imagined or real neglect in the past. Now they feel helpless and excluded. Whatever the reasons, families will compensate for their discomfort by whatever defense mechanism eases their conscience, a process that transfers their discomfort to the personnel of the nursing home. On the other hand, families that fail to visit are employing a mechanism of denial or avoidance, a kind of adjustment by which the patient is, in a sense, dead to them. Thus, they avoid the feeling of guilt that visitation inevitably arouses.

Nurses may encounter some difficulty in understanding some aspects of these problems because, when one of their own family is in the hospital, they may have special privileges and may take part in the care of the relative. They may surmount some of the difficulties of a family situation by considering the family constellation rather than regarding the patient as a separate entity. This implies that they will attempt to understand both the emotional and financial impact of illness upon the family and will realize that relatives who are anxious and sometimes guilt-ridden are entitled to some of the tender loving care that is normally lavished on the patient. In attempting to solve her problems, the nurse can do much to alleviate family distress by maintaining two-way communciation, by making herself reasonably available to the family, and, within reasonable limits, by involving the family in the simple and supplementary aspects of care.

5

The Diabetic Patient

━━━━━◆•◆━━━━━

Diabetes has been known for over 2,000 years. It was accurately described by the Greeks and Romans, although the diagnosis was crude. Because it has been known for so long, one tends to think of diabetes as simply another chronic disease: the patient takes insulin or follows a diet, and that ends the problem. Actually, however, diabetes constitutes one of the most important medical problems in the United States and some European countries.

Incidence

Directly or indirectly, diabetes is now one of the ten leading causes of deaths in the United States, its incidence having more than doubled in the last ten years. One of every 60 persons in the United States has diabetes. The incidence is lower in the Orient and the South Pacific, and higher in Central Europe.

Although the general increase in life expectancy augments the number of persons who acquire the disease in old age and the greater accuracy of diagnosis contributes to a statistical increase, the real basis of the rising incidence of diabetes is to be sought in family backgrounds. Although it is frequently stated that diabetes is familial in nature, but it is not really hereditary, diabetes *is definitely* a hereditary disease. It is transmitted as a recessive trait. In simple terms, a recessive trait is one that cannot appear unless it is inherited from both sides of the family; examples are red hair and blue eyes. A dominant trait such as black hair or brown eyes may be inherited from only one side of a family and yet occur in all of the children.

The recessive diabetic trait, like the red hair-blue eyes combination, may be manifest on both sides of the family, but it is not necessarily present in the same generation. For example, if both parents are diabetic, all the children living to late adulthood will be diabetic; this fact is true even though the parents may not acquire diabetes until very late in life. If one parent is a diabetic and the other carries the trait, 3 of 4 of their children will have diabetes. In a marriage between a diabetic person and one who is nondiabetic and does not have the trait, 50 per cent of the offspring will have the disease. In a family in which both parents possess the diabetic trait and yet neither is diabetic, although their grandparents were, 1 of 4 children will have diabetes. Finally, in a family composed of one parent with a known diabetic trait and one with the trait in the family within three generations, the possibility of diabetes becomes 1 of 7 or 8, or 12.5 per cent.

These are revealing odds. Furthermore, if there is

diabetes within 3 generations and the person is female, overweight, past the menopause, and has had multiple pregnancies, the chances are high that she will become a diabetic. If this potential patient has a baby who weighed 9 pounds or more at birth during one of these pregnancies, her chances are even greater. With a 9-pound baby there is a 75 per cent chance of the mother's becoming a diabetic, regardless of family background. With every pound of birth-weight increase, up to a birth weight of 13 pounds, the risk of diabetes gradually increases until it reaches 100 per cent. These are not general statistics; these are well-documented facts.

There are now at least 3 million persons with diabetes in the United States, and perhaps more. About two-thirds of these are known. The diabetic person is a diabetic, not only when he acquires the typical symptoms—thirst, urinary frequency, and weight loss with a good appetite—but also when he has chemical diabetes, discovered incidentally from a routine test for blood sugar. Chemical diabetes is diabetes; there is no such thing as a little "touch" of diabetes. If one has diabetes, it is immaterial whether it was determined through a glucose tolerance test or through the discovery of massive amounts of glucose in the urine. It does not matter whether the patient is 13 or 109 years old; diabetes has been discovered in babies as young as 6 weeks and in persons over 100 years of age. The juvenile has yet to grow, which makes the disease more difficult to control, but the complications in the juvenile apply equally to the adult. Duration of the disease is the most important fact. If an adult aged 65 has had the disease for 10 or

15 years, he is in as much difficulty as the juvenile of 13 who has had it for 10 or 12 years. They may not be comparable physically, but they are alike in relation to diabetes.

Diagnosis

What can the physician do about diabetes? He cannot modify the hereditary factor, for one cannot change a patient's ancestors. However, the physician can diagnose the condition promptly and accurately and then propose changes in the patient's body weight and in his physical activity, both of which affect tolerance to carbohydrates. The diagnosis will seldom be obvious; it is not very often that one finds symptoms in an elderly adult with newly discovered diabetes unless he has an infection or an injury such as a broken hip. Injury in old people is frequently the precipitating stress that elicits this hereditary trait. People with injuries, burns, or infections of any sort therefore become suspect.

If one wishes to learn that a patient is really a diabetic, a test of a urine specimen obtained at 7 a.m. will not be revealing. A urine specimen about an hour or an hour and a half after he has had a high-carbohyrate meal will be of more significance. If it is negative, then there is a fair possibility that he is not diabetic. If doubt still exists, however, a blood sugar taken at the same time after a meal is a better test. If this is normal, the resulting decision that the patient is nondiabetic is more likely to be accurate. If the blood sugar after a meal is not normal, he has diabetes. If the result is borderline, a glucose tolerance test is necessary. If any one of these tests proves to be positive, the patient has diabetes, provided the diagnosis of abnormality is reproducible.

Symptoms in Old People

William Osler said, "Listen to the patient, and he'll tell you the diagnosis." Although this is true, one must know the signs and symptoms and listen for them. A patient does not diagnose himself as a diabetic; he complains about itching, or needing to have his glasses adjusted after only six months, or being dizzy. General body itching, although not seen often in young people, is a fairly common symptom of diabetes at onset in elderly patients. Another symptom of diabetes, which is probably commoner but not very often mentioned in books, is what many patients call dizziness. Response to close questioning reveals that the dizziness is neither vertigo nor spinning, but a strange, lightheaded feeling, a sensation that the head is two feet above the shoulders. After questioning, patients often recognize the difference and will use the more descriptive term, "floating." There is no therapy for some types of dizziness, but there is a very specific therapy for the dizziness of chemical diabetes.

One of the first symptoms of diabetes in an elderly patient may be lack of sensation in the feet. On examination, the feet may show signs of poor circulation, often with ulceration. Additionally, if the patient's glasses must be changed every six months and if he notices a frequent shifting of the position of the newspaper or book, one should suspect diabetes. Distance vision may also be changing constantly—a symptom of glaucoma which is a frequent finding in elderly diabetic patients. This, too, should be considered and investigated.

Treatment

Once the diagnosis of diabetes is made, treatment should be instituted promptly, whatever the patient's age. Active treatment means attention to the basic principles of diet; the administration of insulin or oral hypoglycemic agents, if necessary; and exercise within the patient's limitations.

EXERCISE

Exercise, obviously, will be very limited in elderly people confined to chronic-disease hospitals and nursing homes, but it is feasible. Walking should be prescribed to the physically able. Very often in such institutions, however, walking the patient down the hall six or seven times a day is considered an inconvenient chore. Although the effort is time-consuming and seemingly minor, it is nevertheless important.

DIET

When a doctor diagnoses diabetes in a nursing-home patient, the staff despairs and envisages a complicated diet that must be calculated, measured, and weighed. They can be reassured, however, by the American Diabetic Association exchange list, with the figures given very simply, without resorting to arithmetic; they can quickly learn to use the slide rule that comes with the booklets and can easily be taught the use of a teaspoon, a tablespoon, and a measuring cup as measuring instruments. After a short time, any untrained, intelligent kitchen helper becomes proficient in measuring with such simple tools and is able to evolve a fairly accurate measured diet that is reasonable for a particular diabetic patient whose intake must be measured.

The diabetic diet merely excludes sugars and sweets. Other factors are important. A patient, for example, may be eating six slices of bread a day and really require only four. I recall an elderly patient whose diabetes became acute with an infection. When the infection was improving, the patient went to a nursing home; a painstaking nursing supervisor made him follow his diet conscientiously. Although he once required 60 units of insulin to control his diabetes, he now requires no insulin for the control of the disease. Thanks to the nurse's care in measuring the unweighed prescribed diet, he does not even require an oral hypoglycemic agent. Such management is possible and it is important. This aspect of care cannot be overstressed. The exchange system and exchange lists are given at the end of the chapter.

WEIGHT

Another point to be stressed in the treatment of diabetes is the patient's weight. Before prescribing hypoglycemic agents and insulin, the patient's weight must be considered. At least eight out of ten persons with diabetes are overweight at onset. Giving insulin or tolbutamide (Orinase) initially, unless there is infection or some other precipitating factor, is often a mistake. A diet to ensure a weight loss averaging a pound a week controls the disease in more than 90 per cent of the overweight group. The other 20 per cent of diabetic patients are usually thin or underweight, but still may not be controlled by diet alone. Their blood sugars remain high, with or without sugar in the urine, and they need additional treatment. If they have no small blood vessel complications (that is, eye or kidney trouble), oral hypoglycemic agents can be used if they prove effective. The patient with small blood vessel disease should not be given oral agents. He may require only 6 or 8 units of insulin, but this is far safer than using an oral agent. We know what insulin can do; we are not as yet sufficiently acquainted with the effects of oral agents.

FOOT CARE

In addition to general care, one must not overlook the care of the feet. When the first evidence of gangrene or the first infected ulcer appears, or when the first midthigh guillotine-type amputation is required, it is too late. Just as diabetic coma and acidosis theoretically are totally avoidable, the foot and lower-extremity complications in diabetes are generally preventable. Almost invariably these so-called accidents are not "accidents." They involve a combination of factors. The diabetic patient feels very little with his feet; he has neuropathy and neuritis, does not sense temperatures, and often feels no pain. As a matter of fact, an elderly diabetic patient may have neuritis, numbness, and lack of sensation in the feet as a first symptom. Neuropathy is not a long-term complication. The main complications result from poor circulation, the lack of sensation for heat and cold (especially heat), and for surface pain—that is, the pain one feels when stuck with a needle, not the pain of a hard irregular surface such as that of walking on a rocky driveway. Consequently, the diabetic patient, walking in ill-fitting shoes, cloth slippers, or barefooted, may experience a little crack or abrasion without being aware of the injury, and consequently suffers an infection. Although the elderly patient should inspect his feet, he is often too old to do so or know what to look for. It is the nurse's responsibility to check the feet, a procedure that takes only a few minutes. A brief examination of the feet at least once a day to make certain that no new crack or abrasion has appeared is important. A piece of glass the size of a pinhead can cause an ulcer on the toe in a diabetic patient. When an abrasion or cut occurs, the patient must relieve the foot of all weight; no matter how minor the injury, there must be no weight bearing and no walking. Only by such treatment can one improve circulation and rest the affected part. The doctor should be notified promptly. In general, therapy is the same as that for any infection: antibiotics, local hygienic treatment, removal of the foreign body, or other indicated procedure.

The statement that cleanliness is of prime importance is especially applicable to the feet of diabetics. Adults constantly pick up dirt and dust through the seams of the shoes. Daily bathing, drying, and avoidance of such secondary infections as athlete's foot may seem to be minor chores, but the neglect of these services leads to massive cellulitis in the diabetic patient who has poor circulation, neuritis, and lack of sensation. Such neglect may lead to surgical problems. Although nurses may realize that this can occur, only observation of the end-results of a minor scratch, perhaps involving amputation, can demonstrate that a seemingly minor abrasion can be the cause of a really serious disability. Then the patient who is unable to master crutches and cannot manage a prosthetic limb becomes a bed patient, with all of the attending problems. Obviously, neglect can cause additional work for nurses and misery for the patient.

Recent Developments in Diabetes

There is definite hope for improvement in the treatment of diabetes. Although new treatments for cancer, leukemia, and heart disease are dramatized, one hears little about discoveries in the treatment of diabetes. In the last year, for example, "human insulin" has been made from hog insulin by removing one small chemical group from the end of the formula. The product has not yet been marketed, but the material has been used in diabetic patients who are insulin-resistant. This is an important discovery; some patients who once required thousands of units of insulin, often because they had unusual levels of insulin antibodies, now manage on 8, 10, or 15 units of this manufactured insulin. Several researchers independently synthesized the opposite halves of the human insulin molecule from raw chemicals; the resultant A and B chains were attached to the opposite chains of hog insulin. When this product was injected into animals, it lowered blood sugar. When the two synthetic chains were joined, the substance did not perform as well as commercial insulin, although it was still insulin. Although some group is missing, there is hope that soon we shall have a synthetic man-made insulin. Although it will not cure diabetes, it may make a vast difference in both the degree and the ease of control and will be an accomplishment almost as great as that of the original discovery of insulin. In preinsulin days, juveniles lived an average of 11 months and adults about 27 months after the diagnosis was made. Juveniles now live an average of two-thirds of a normal life span; adults, depending on age of onset, live almost a normal life expectancy. The statistics are encouraging even with our present elementary resources; new discoveries point to even more dramatic successes.

One factor that is not very hopeful is that diabetes is a growing disease. We can almost never control the spread of diabetes as we can that of an infectious disease, because it is futile to advise a young juvenile diabetic not to marry a girl whose grandmother had diabetes. We can now experimentally control genetics in some lower animals and plants to change hereditary transmission characteristics. If this is possible in plants and fruit flies, we can hope that it may eventually be possible in other areas. The research in progress, the increasing interest of the medical profession and the public, and progress in the treatment of diabetes in the last fifteen years all give hope that dramatic developments in this area still lie ahead. We shall achieve practicable and more effective methods of prevention. In the view of some, it is not too much to hope for the discovery of a cure for diabetes mellitus.

The Exchange System for Diabetic Diets*

There are a number of ways to plan diabetic diets. The easiest one is the Exchange System, in which sim-

*Adapted from *Diet Manual for Long Term Medical Care Facilities.* Hospitals Section, Hartford: Connecticut State Department of Health, 1964.

ilar foods are grouped together into six substitution lists to form the milk, vegetable, fruit, bread, meat, and fat exchanges, as indicated on the following pages. Individual diets are planned on the basis of the number of "exchanges" from each list allowed during the day. One serving from each group is called an exchange. Thus,

$$1 \text{ small orange} = 1 \text{ fruit exchange}$$
$$1 \text{ slice bacon} = 1 \text{ fat exchange}$$

The size of the serving is important. Remember that each serving is one exchange. If the serving is doubled it equals two exchanges:

$$1 \text{ slice bread} = 1 \text{ bread exchange}$$
$$2 \text{ slices bread} = 2 \text{ bread exchanges}$$

Foods within each list may be exchanged for one another. For example:

1 bread exchange = 1 slice bread, 1 small potato, 1 muffin, or ½ cup cooked cereal

Generally speaking, foods from one group may not be substituted for foods from another group. In other words, one cannot make one fruit exchange for one meat exchange. A few exceptions to this are noted on the Exchange Lists. No others should be made except by one who knows how to calculate food values.

These exchange lists were developed to provide variety in the diet. They are not in themselves a diet. The physician will prescribe the amounts or number of each of the exchanges that may be allowed each day.

Certain seasonings and food items listed below may be used as desired in the preparation of meals:

Chopped parsley	Mint
Garlic	Onion
Celery	Nutmeg
Mustard	Cinnamon
Pepper and other spices	Saccharin or Sucaryl
Lemon	Vinegar

The following items have practically no food value and may also be used as desired:

Coffee	Rennet tablets
Tea	Pickles, sour
Clear broth	Pickles, unsweetened dill
Bouillon, without fat	Cranberries
Gelatin, unsweetened	Rhubarb

TABLE 1

Milk Exchanges

One milk exchange contains carbohydrate 12 grams, protein 8 grams, fat 10 grams = 170 calories.*

	Amount
Whole milk (plain or homogenized)	1 cup
Skim milk	1 cup
Evaporated milk	½ cup
Powdered whole milk	¼ cup
Powdered skim milk (nonfat dried milk)	¼ cup
Buttermilk (made from whole milk)	1 cup
Buttermilk (made from skim milk)	1 cup

* Skim milk products contain less fat. When exchanging for whole milk, add two fat exchanges to get the same food value.

TABLE 2
Vegetable Exchanges

Vegetable Exchanges A. These contain negligible amounts of carbohydrate, protein, and fat. In raw form, size of serving unlimited; cooked, size of serving ½ to 1 cup.

Asparagus	Greens:*
Broccoli	beet greens
Brussels sprouts*	chard
Cabbage	collards
Cauliflower	dandelion
Celery	kale
Chicory*	mustard
Cucumber	spinach
Escarole*	turnip greens
Eggplant	Sauerkraut
Lettuce	String beans, young
Mushrooms	Summer squash
Okra	Tomatoes*
Green pepper*	Watercress*
Radishes*	

Vegetable Exchanges B. These contain carbohydrate 7 grams, protein 2 grams = 35 calories. One serving equals ½ cup.

Beets	Pumpkin
Carrots*	Rutabagas
Onions	Squash, winter*
Peas, green	Turnips

---

* Contains a considerable amount of vitamin A.

TABLE 3

Fruit Exchanges

One fruit exchange contains carbohydrate 10 grams = 40 calories. Fruits may be fresh, dried, cooked, canned, or frozen, provided no sugar is added.

	Amount		Amount
Apple			
(2 in. diam.)	1 small	Grapes	12
Applesauce	½ cup	Grape juice	¼ cup
Apricots, fresh	2 medium	Honeydew, medium	⅛
Apricots, dried	4½ small	Mango	½ small
Banana	½ small	Orange*	1 small
Blackberries	1 cup	Orange juice*	½ cup
Raspberries	1 cup	Papaya	⅓ medium
Strawberries*	1 cup	Peach	1 medium
Blueberries	⅔ cup	Pear	1 small
Cantaloupe*	¼	Pineapple	½ cup
(6 in. diam.)			
Cherries	10 large	Pineapple juice	⅓ cup
Dates	2	Plums	2 medium
Figs, fresh	2 large	Prunes, dried	2 medium
Figs, dried	1 small	Raisins	2 tablespoons
Grapefruit *	½ small	Tangerine*	1 large
Grapefruit juice*	½ cup	Watermelon	1 cup

* Contains a considerable amount of vitamin C (ascorbic acid).

TABLE 4

Bread Exchanges

One bread exchange contains carbohydrate 15 grams, protein 2 grams = 70 calories.

	Amount
Bread	1 slice
biscuit, roll (2 in. diam.)	1
muffin (2 in. diam.)	1
cornbread (1½ in. cu.)	1
Cereals, cooked	½ cup
dry, flake, and puff types	¾ cup
Rice, grits, cooked	½ cup
Spaghetti, noodles, cooked	½ cup
Macaroni, cooked	½ cup
Crackers	
graham (2½ in. sq.)	2
oysterettes (½ cup)	20
saltines (2 in. sq.)	5
soda (2½ in. sq.)	3
round, thin	6
Flour	2½ tablespoons
Vegetables	
beans and peas, dried, cooked (lima, navy, split peas, cowpea, etc.)	½ cup
baked beans, no pork, molasses, or sugar	¼ cup
corn	1 cup
popcorn	1 cup
parsnips	⅔ cup
Potatoes	
white	1 small
potatoes, white, mashed	½ cup
potatoes, sweet, or yams	¼ cup
Sponge cake, plain (1½ in. cu.)	1
Ice cream (omit 2 fat exchanges)	½ cup

TABLE 5

Meat Exchanges

One meat exchange contains protein 7 grams, fat 5 grams = 75 calories. Allow 3 meat exchanges for an average-size serving. This is about the same as 2 meatballs, or a small steak (¼ pound raw weight), or 3 of any of the foods listed below.

	Amount
Meat and poultry (medium fat):	
beef, lamb, pork, liver, chicken, etc.	1 ounce
Cold cuts (4½ x ⅛ in.):	
salami, minced ham, bologna, liverwurst, luncheon loaf	1 slice
Frankfurter (8 to 9 per pound)	1
Egg	1
Fish	
haddock, flounder, bass, etc.	1 ounce
salmon, tuna, crab, lobster	¼ cup
shrimps, clams, oysters, etc.	5 small
sardines	3 medium
Cheese	
cheddar type	1 ounce
cottage	¼ cup
Peanut butter	2 tablespoons

TABLE 6

Fat Exchanges

One fat exchange contains fat 5 grams = 45 calories.

	Amount
Butter, margarine	1 teaspoon
Bacon, crisp	1 slice
Cream, light	2 tablespoons
Cream, heavy	1 tablespoon
Cream cheese	1 tablespoon
Avocado (4 in. diam.)	⅛
French dressing	1 tablespoon
Mayonnaise	1 teaspoon
Oil or cooking fat	1 teaspoon
Nuts	6 small
Olives	5 small

6

The Patient with Heart Disease

-------◆◆◆-------

MANY patients in nursing homes already have heart disease; some develop heart failure during their stay. Since this is a condition that readily responds to treatment, it is necessary that registered nurses, practical nurses, and nurses' aides who are in constant attendance on the patients be able to recognize the early symptoms and signs. Early recognition of impending difficulties is most important so that corrective procedures may be started. In a heart that is already damaged, early treatment may make the difference between death and recovery for a patient. It is far better to treat the early signs than to wait until the heart is acutely embarrassed.

Anatomical Review

It is helpful to review the elemental anatomy of the circulatory system, since nearly all congestive failure is due to stoppage of blood flow somewhere in the system of vessels that carry the blood through the body (Figure 1). Starting with the left ventricle, the blood goes through the aortic valve into the aorta and is distributed to the body, head, and extremities. When it enters the tissue spaces, the blood rids itself of oxygen and takes in carbon dioxide, lactic acid, and other end-products before returning to the heart by way of the venous system. The venous blood enters the right atrium from the superior and inferior vena cava, courses through the tricuspid valve into the right ventricle and then through the pulmonary valve and the pulmonary artery (the only place in the body where an artery carries deoxygenated blood) into the lungs. Here carbon dioxide is given off and oxygen is picked up by the blood as one breathes. Finally, the blood enters the pulmonary veins (the only place in the body where the veins carry oxygenated blood) and passes into the left atrium, through the mitral valve, and into the left ventricle.

Any circulatory catastrophe affecting the heart can be fully explained in relation either to this cycle or to interruption of the coronary circulation. In a man who has a thrombosis in the wall of a coronary vessel, the blood supply is shut off to the heart muscle beyond. This is called the area of coronary infarction. Degeneration of the infarcted muscle wall occurs, and the contracting ventricle is weakened.

Types of Congestive Heart Failure

In congestive heart failure, the pumping mechanism of the heart cannot take care of the blood that is offered

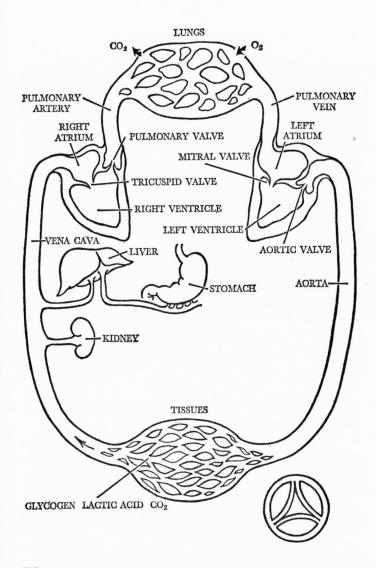

FIG. 1

Cycle of circulation. The heart valves as shown are simplified. The inset of the valves in cross section is a more accurate illustration of their three cusps.

to it. There are two kinds of failure. In the first, the cardiac output is either normal or increased. This occurs in hyperthyroidism, severe anemia, and beriberi or vitamin B_1 deficiency. In hyperthyroidism, the heart may be normal; the body's thermostat is up, causing the tissues to demand more oxygen. The heart, therefore, beats rapidly until finally it tires, and heart failure develops. With anemia, the blood is too "thin"—that is, there are insufficient red blood cells to carry the oxygen, and the heart pumps abnormally, trying to deliver enough oxygenated blood to the tissues. If it pumps too rapidly for too long a period, it fails. The second type of failure occurs with a decreased cardiac output—for example, after a coronary thrombosis or with cardiac arrhythmia. In beriberi there is a dilation of the blood vessels, with a resultant fall in blood pressure; this causes the heart to beat rapidly from reflex reaction. In these circumstances, heart failure can be sudden.

Certain occurrences during cardiac failure add to the problem. First, there is an increase of plasma volume, and second, the ability of the kidney to excrete sodium is decreased. Sodium and water are combined in the body; when the kidney does not excrete sodium adequately, it holds water, and the patient then becomes waterlogged. In cardiac failure, the adrenal glands frequently produce an excess of aldosterone, an adrenal hormone that also serves to hold water in the body. In addition, the permeability of the capillaries is increased so that there is increased flow of water into the tissues, and swelling (edema) occurs.

Congestive heart failure is further divided into left ventricular failure and right ventricular failure. It is useful to understand the difference because the symp-

toms and treatment of these two conditions are some-
what different.

LEFT VENTRICULAR FAILURE

Failure of the left ventricle results in congestion of
the lungs. It is usually acute and sudden, although it
may be preceded by premonitory symptoms. The patient may notice that he puffs on moderate activity.
If, however, he becomes too active and does more than
he should, or if he has eaten too much salt, he begins
to wheeze; to him it appears to be bronchitis. He puffs
as he walks, tires easily, and must sit down. These
early symptoms may resemble those of mild bronchial
asthma.

Causes of Left Ventricular Failure. There are many
causes. In hypertension, due to sclerosis of the arteries
and arterioles in the kidney and throughout the body,
the left ventricle must exert more pressure to push the
blood through the arterioles. The left ventricle, which
is the chief muscle of the heart, thus carries an increased work load and enlarges (ventricular hyper-
trophy) as any exercised muscle does. Eventually the left
ventricle tires and is unable to handle the blood deliv-
ered to it by the relatively normal right ventricle. Then
blood backs up, and fluid accumulates in the lungs.

In coronary disease, which in elderly patients is
caused by sclerosis of the coronary vessels, there is often
a sudden plugging (thrombosis) of a coronary artery,
with damage to the heart mucle (myocardial infarction)
beyond the plug (thrombus). If the left ventricle is
injured with consequent weakening of its contraction,
left ventricular failure develops. If the atrio-ventricu-

lar node, the bundle of His or its branches are affected, cardiac arrhythmia may develop and in turn cause heart failure. This is discussed later.

AORTIC VALVE. Disease of the aortic valve of the heart can lead to ventricular fatigue and decompensation. In rheumatic fever the valve may become scarred and unable to close, causing aortic regurgitation or insufficiency. If the valve is scarred open, it resembles a defective bicycle tire pump—that is, the gasket is worn, air escapes, and more pumping is required to fill the tire with air. The ventricle pushes the blood through the aortic valve; because the aortic valve does not close, however, blood flows back through the valve. It therefore requires more pumping action to push the blood out into the body tissues. Finally, the heart fails very rapidly. The aortic valve may also be narrowed because of scar tissue and calcium. The aortic-valve opening, which should be the size of a silver dollar, may be narrowed by calcium deposits and scar tissue down to less than the diameter of a pencil lead. The left ventricle, trying to push blood through a small opening, gradually becomes enlarged and finally weakens.

MITRAL VALVE. Mitral insufficiency, which also causes left-sided heart failure, means that the mitral valve between the left atrium and the left ventricle is scarred open. In this case the left ventricle contracts and sends the blood through to the aorta; since the mitral valve does not close completely, some blood flows back into the left atrium, making the left ventricle's pumping action inefficient. This inefficiency results in an increased work load on the left ventricle and ultimately causes left ventricular failure.

ARRHYTHMIA. Arrhythmia or irregular rhythms can cause heart failure. In atrial fibrillation, the atria may beat at a rate of 300 per minute, while the ventricle may have a rate of 80 to 160 beats per minute. Rapid atrial fibrillation may lead to failure. Atrial flutter occurs, for example, when the atria are beating at a rate of 250 and the ventricles at a rate of 125 per minute; this is known as a 2 : 1 block. In ventricular tachycardia, there is an extremely rapid ventricular rhythm, running from 120 to 200 beats per minute. Ventricular tachycardia usually is caused by too much digitalis. Unfortunately, sometimes the patient is believed to need more digitalis, and more is given, which makes a bad situation worse.

OTHER CAUSES. Inflammation of the myocardium or muscle of the heart is called myocarditis. It is caused by virus diseases such as influenza. Old tissue slides from the influenza epidemics of 1918 and 1920, recently examined, show the same changes as those of the virus myocarditis of today. The myocardial changes in rheumatic fever are not due to the infection itself, but to an allergy to the infection—that is, an inflammation that causes a weakening of the muscle fibers and failure. Some now rare diseases such as typhoid and diphtheria also cause myocarditis. In subacute bacterial endocarditis the heart valves are destroyed by infection. These inflammations may cause congestive heart failure.

Signs and Symptoms. The first symptoms of left ventricular failure are shortness of breath (dyspnea), with wheezing and coughing. Occasionally this occurs in paroxysms at night: the patient wakes up gasping for breath, goes over to the window, takes a few breaths, and then sits on the edge of the bed for 15 minutes before feeling able to lie down and sleep. The patient also may be unable to lie flat and breathe comfortably (orthopnea). Anxiety develops; the patient knows that something is seriously wrong; he has a feeling of impending doom and is restless. The signs of left ventricular failure are cyanosis of the nails and the lips; there may be sweating, and the skin is pale and cold. There will be a rapid heart beat (tachycardia); a gallop rhythm may also develop. This is pathognomonic of left ventricular failure. If one listens with a stethoscope over the precordium, one will hear a rhythm like the gallop of a horse. Gallop rhythm is ominous and indicates impending pulmonary edema and severe failure. It must be treated immediately, and the physician must be called at once.

RIGHT VENTRICULAR FAILURE

Failure of the right ventricle leads to congestion of the venous systems and exudation of fluid from the serous surfaces that line the chest and the abdominal walls. Usually this type of failure develops more slowly than left-sided failure.

Causes. This condition arises when there is interference with the flow of blood through the pulmonary system. The interference may result from pulmonary hypertension, pulmonary stenosis, or pulmonary emboli. Congenital defects also can interfere with the normal flow of blood to the lungs. When there is systemic congestion of both the left and the right sides of the heart, the term "congestive heart failure" is preferred. Thus, when mitral disease or other left-sided injury causes both left-sided and right-sided failure, this term should be used.

In right-sided failure there is a blockage either in the pulmonary artery or the pulmonary bed. The right ventricle must push blood through a narrowed artery or through a lung field blocked by previous pulmonary emboli. The right ventricle becomes overstretched and overstrained. Ultimately, it is unable to pump the blood that is returned to it, and there is a back-up of blood, causing congestion of the liver and kidneys and generalized edema.

The signs of right-sided heart failure are as follows. First, there is cyanosis, which is general. Second, there is distention of the neck veins with the patient in the sitting position. A person lying down may have distended neck veins, but if they remain distended when the person sits up, it means that the blood cannot flow up to the heart, even with the help of gravity; something is blocking it. Also, if the arm is raised and the veins are still distended, the normal venous return is being blocked. Third, fluid collects in the chest as pleural fluid and in the abdomen as ascites. Fourth, the ankles and the feet of a person with severe right ventricular failure are swollen with edema. The liver is enlarged and congested; jaundice is present only with severe liver congestion. Because of the enlarged liver and congested stomach, there are symptoms of anorexia, nausea, and a slight jaundice.

Treatment

When the signs or symptoms of congestive heart failure first appear in a patient, the nursing supervisor or head nurse on duty should be informed immediately.

She, in turn, should notify the physician-in-charge. Only a physician should treat the acute cause of heart failure.

ACUTE LEFT VENTRICULAR FAILURE

Acute left ventricular failure causing pulmonary edema is a medical emergency. Treatment of this condition may begin with the treatment of paroxysmal nocturnal dyspnea. One night the patient may have acute dyspnea, and the nurse may find him sitting on the edge of the bed or lying flat in bed, gasping, anxious, and restless. Rales may be heard in his lungs. The patient will demand to sit up; he cannot lie flat. When the patient sits up, he reduces the volume of blood in the lungs by 500 ml. or one pint. This increases his lung capacity. Therefore, the first thing to do is put him in a bed in a true Fowler's position—that is, the head of the bed is raised 18 to 20 inches—or place him in a chair. He should have oxygen, usually under positive pressure. The physician-in-charge should be notified as soon as possible, especially if this the first episode. Morphine or meperidine hydrochloride (Demorol) should be given under doctor's orders to allay the anxiety, which itself causes rapid respiration; 1/6 grain or even 1/4 grain of morphine may be given if the patient is in really poor condition. Tourniquets are useful in dealing with congestion in the lung. Since the right side of the heart continues to push blood into the already congested lungs, to give the patient relief, the venous return is decreased by placing tourniquets on three of the four extremities and then rotating them.

If the patient has not been receiving digitalis, it should be given, usually by vein. A diuretic may also be given, although it will not work in less than four to six hours. Aminophylline should be given, particularly if it is uncertain whether the wheezing is due to bronchial asthma or to heart failure. Aminophylline is a bronchial dilator, a mild diuretic, and a respiratory and myocardial stimulant; it is a good drug to use, except in the rare case when the subject is hypersensitive to it. Once a patient has recovered from an episode of left ventricular failure, he should be treated as having had chronic heart failure and should be started on a low-salt diet with appropriate drug therapy. This will be considered later.

ACUTE RIGHT VENTRICULAR FAILURE

The treatment of severe right ventricular failure involves placing the patient in Fowler's position, the exact position depending on the degree of dyspnea. Oxygen is given to aid breathing. The physician-in-charge should be notified. He may remove some of the fluid in the chest by thoracentesis or that in the abdomen by paracentesis. Proper digitalization is indicated, since patients who are in failure may well be underdigitalized. Diuretics will be used routinely, and here the low-salt diet is of extreme importance. After the patient's condition has been stabilized, he should be started on the proper regimen for a patient with chronic heart failure.

CHRONIC HEART FAILURE

The physician must closely follow the cardiac patient who is on medication to regulate and supervise activity, diet, and medication. The responsibility for carrying out the doctor's orders and for reporting the effects of medication on the patient lies with the nurse. Untoward drug reactions and the signs of digitalis toxicity should be immediately reported to the physician.

ACTIVITY

Bed rest favors diuresis; chair rest helps pulmonary edema but increases the peripheral edema. In cases of chronic failure, one attempts to strike a happy medium. Keep the patient up in the morning and put him to bed in the late afternoon, at which time diuresis will occur. The patient with chronic cardiac disease should be allowed to walk to the bathroom; this will help to prevent the occurrence of pulmonary emboli. Slow ambulation around a room hurts no one except the patient with a recent coronary and possible rupture of the ventricle. Too many patients are kept in bed. Such a regimen may result only in filling their lungs and their abdomens with fluid. These patients should be kept ambulant; when this is not possible, they can at least be moved and turned frequently.

DIET

These patients should receive a salt-free diet. Although various diets are low in salt, the severely ill cardiac patient should be on salt-free bread and salt-free milk as well. Food should be dusted with salt in the kitchen. The cardiac patient must learn to sprinkle a little lemon or onion juice on his food or use a salt substitute. The diet should be low in salt, starches, and fats and contain adequate amounts of protein. Vitamin supplements are often indicated in nursing-home diets.

DRUGS

Much is still unknown about digitalis and its action. The proper doses for digitalization and maintenance cannot be stated exactly because the requirement varies from patient to patient. Some patients do well in treatment of cardiac failure on 0.1 mg of digitoxin three times a week. If 0.5 mg of digitoxin are given per week, such a patient may go into digitalis intoxication, whereas another patient may take 0.3 mg of digitoxin every day and digest it with no difficulty. The optimum dose of digitalis, then, is that which gives the patient optimum improvement—that is, diuresis and relief of symptoms of congestive failure. Once the physician has prescribed digitalis, the nurse must watch for signs of overdigitalization or underdigitalization by pulse, by clinical appearance, by weight, and by tests of the vital capacity. If the patient has a morning pulse of 54 and does well throughout the rest of the day, he is receiving the proper dosage. The signs of digitalis intoxication are loss of appetite, nausea and vomiting, diarrhea, disturbances in vision, and mental confusion. The pulse may reveal some ectopic beats—that is, extra beats followed by a long pause. In digitalis intoxication there is bigeminy, a premature beat coupled with each normal beat. The patient may feel poor; he may actually show shortness of breath with all these irregularities. Ventricular tachycardia—the ventricle beating at a rate of about 160—may develop. This is a dangerous condition that requires immediate hospital treatment.

Overdigitalization is treated by stopping the digitalis. If the heart then goes into failure, potassium can be given. Potassium chloride is irritating, but it can be given in a syrup form as Potassium Triplex. Potassium may be furnished by giving a full glass of orange juice each day or salt-free bouillon twice a day; this obviates the need for a pill or an expensive syrup. Reducing the potassium level by diuresis increases the danger of digitalis toxicity from a "normal" dose of digitalis. Again, should signs of digitalis toxicity appear, potassium should be given in orange juice or bouillon or as potassium chloride, if this is well tolerated. Diuretics should be discontinued as soon as they are not needed.

7

Indication and Use of
Modern Drugs

---·•·---

E VERY drug is a chemical and has some potential
for harm. It will be useful therapeutically only when
given in the correct dose, for an appropriate condition,
for an optimal period, and by the best route of administration. An understanding of the mechanism of drug
action, of side-effects, and of drug interactions will add
to the efficacy of the treatment and help to improve
patient care.

It is generally wise to be neither the first nor the
last to use a new drug unless one is engaged in research.
So many new drugs are released after limited testing
that idiosyncratic reactions often cannot be evaluated
in the trials. This is not an indictment of the ethical
drug houses which are generally careful, but rather an
admission of the fact that one cannot make predictions
from small samples. Thalidomide was tested exhaus-
tively in animals and found to be remarkably safe. It
was used in Europe for four years before its shocking
effects were discovered.

With the thousands of drugs available for prescription use, several thousand proprietary names tend to confuse the medical profession. It is best to learn and use the generic name of drugs whenever possible. There is often a monetary saving in ordering a drug by its generic name. Sources of unbiased information on new drugs are scarce. Books that can be recommended include:

1. *New and Nonofficial Drugs.* Philadelphia: J. B. Lippincott Co. This has been published yearly by the A.M.A. Council on Drugs, but is to be replaced soon by a new publication called *New Drugs.*
2. *Drugs of Choice.* St. Louis: C. V. Mosby Co. Edited by Walter Modell, this book is published biennially.
3. *Current Therapy.* Philadelphia: W. B. Saunders Co., 1966. Edited by Howard F. Conn and revised annually.

These books are written by panels of experts and are reliable. A useful compilation of information about drugs is available in the *Physicians' Desk Reference,* which is distributed to doctors every year by Medical Economics, Inc. The information is accurate, but not unbiased, since it is supplied by the drug houses.

Current medical journals are a good source of information, but the relevant articles are generally scattered. *The New England Journal of Medicine* publishes at frequent intervals a brief but highly informative series of articles entitled "Current Concepts in Therapy." These are written by experts and are reliable. A very fine journal called *The Medical Letter on Drugs and Thera-*

peutics is published biweekly by Drugs and Therapeutics Information, Inc., 305 East 45th St., New York, N.Y. Devoted exclusively to an apprasial of modern drugs, this publication is of an unusually high caliber and should be on the shelf of every physician and available in every medical library, hospital, and nursing home. Any administrator would perform a service to his staff by making *The Medical Letter* available. It will improve drug therapy and thereby enhance the quality of patient care.

Antimicrobial Drugs

ANTIBIOTICS

In choosing drugs for the treatment of infectious diseases, one is essentially engaging in a search for agents with selective toxicity. A chemical is required that will injure or destroy the essential life process in the microorganism while exerting little or no toxic effect on the host, the patient. The search for such a "magic bullet" began with Paul Ehrlich around the turn of the century and led to his discovery of salvarsan ("606"). Thereafter, not much progress was made until Sir Alexander Fleming's fortuitous observation of the effect of the mold *Penicillium notatum* on bacterial cultures in 1929. This discovery was not exploited for therapy until 10 years later, when Howard W. Florey and Ernest Boris Chain demonstrated the feasibility of growing the mold and extracting and purifying the active antibiotic substance for the treatment of human disease. The success of this approach inspired Selman Waksman and his colleagues to reexplore the antibiotic potential of the *Actinomyces* species from which streptomycin and a host of other antibiotics have been obtained. The development and widespread use of antibiotics has been the most important single advance in medicine since the days of Pasteur, Koch, and Ehrlich. Familiarity with antibiotics is a daily necessity for all persons caring for sick patients.

Penicillin. The original penicillin and the prototype to which all other derivatives should be compared is benzyl penicillin (penicillin G). This compound is isolated directly from the mold and is most active against Gram-positive bacteria, especially *Pneumococcus, Streptococcus,* and *Staphylococcus,* and also against the Gram-negative *Gonococcus* and *Meningococcus,* the spirochete of syphilis, some of the *Actinomyces,* and some of the larger viruses such as those causing trachoma and lymphogranuloma venereum. With long use, however, many *Staphylococci* have now become resistant to penicillin. In the vast majority of cases, this is due to the action of the enzyme penicillinase made by some strains of *Staphylococcus.*

Pencillin exerts some of its effects by blocking synthesis of the bacterial cell wall. This leaves the bacterium susceptible to destruction, but does not injure the animal cell because it has no cell wall, only a cell membrane. This is a prime example of selective toxicity. For all practical purposes, there is no toxic dose of penicillin, and its dangers all accrue from its potential to sensitize patients for immunological sequelae—for example, rash, dermatitis, anaphylaxis, and serum sickness.

The usual form of penicillin is the sodium or potassium salt of benzyl penicillin, more commonly known as penicillin G. It is dispensed as 125-mg tablets (200,-000 units) or multiples thereof for oral use or as a syrup for pediatric use. Parenteral preparations include aqueous penicillin G for intravenous use or procaine penicillin for intramuscular use. A particularly long-acting form is benzathine penicillin (Bicillin), which is injected intramuscularly and gives detectable blood levels for 2 to 4 weeks, depending on the dose used.

Although penicillin G has been and is used extensively for oral therapy, it is acid-labile, and a very significant proportion, perhaps 50 per cent is destroyed by gastric acid, so that only 25 to 35 per cent of an oral dose is actually absorbed. Thus, to achieve adequate blood levels, very high doses must be used. To obviate this problem phenoxymethyl penicillin (Penicillin V, V-Cillin, Pen-Vee, and Compocillin) and phenethicillin (Syncillin, Duracillin, and Maxipen) were developed. These modified penicillins are acid-stable and are well absorbed from the gastrointestinal tract; a 250-mg (400,000-unit) tablet of one of these preparations will give a blood level similar to that resulting from 187 mg (300,000 units) of intramuscular procaine penicillin. The antibacterial spectrum of these modified penicillins is identical to that of penicillin G. However, many strains of *Staphylococcus* now produce penicillinase and are completely resistant to the previously mentioned penicillin preparations. These resistant strains now represent at least 50 per cent of the staphylococcal infections acquired in hospitals and are responsible for a significant mortality. In former years, this meant that one was compelled to change to other antibiotics to which the resistant *Staphylococcus* might respond.

Very recently, chemists have succeeded in splitting the benzyl penicillin molecule to 6-aminopenicillinic acid and then attaching new side chains to it to produce a large variety of new semisynthetic penicillins. Those that have been marketed are listed in Table 1, which also indicates some of their significant properties. Sodium methicillin was the first to demonstrate an effect on the penicillin-resistant *Staphylococcus* and has had the most use. It must be given by injection because it is labile to gastric acid. The usual adult dose is 1 gm every 4 to 6 hours. Recently, sodium oxacillin has become available for both oral and parenteral use; it appears to be more potent. The usual adult dose is 0.25 to 0.5 gm 4 times a day. As this is written, sodium oxacillin is being released for general use, and experience with it is limited. One would suppose that it will follow the pattern of sodium oxacillin in most or all respects. Sodium nafcillin can be used orally or parenterally with a dosage schedule identical to that of sodium oxacillin, since it is also acid-stable and effective against penicillin-resistant staphylococci.

A spectacular advance in therapy has resulted from the semisynthetic sodium ampicillin. This drug has an increased spectrum of antibacterial activity and is effective against many Gram-negative bacteria including *Escherichia coli, Hemophilus influenzae, Neisseria gonorrhoeae, Neisseria meningitidis, Brucella melitensis, Brucella abortus, Proteus mirabilis,* and many strains of *Salmonella* and *Shigella.* It is acid-stable and at present is given orally; however, a parenteral preparation has proved to be safe and effective and should be approved by the Food and Drug Administration before this material is in print. It should be noted that sodium ampicillin is penicillinase-labile and therefore is useless against penicillin-resistant staphylococci. The usual adult dose is 250 to 500 mg 4 times a day.

TABLE 1

The Penicillins and Their Properties*

Group	Generic Name	Trade Names	Acid-	Penicillinase-
Benzyl	penicillin G	many	Labile	Labile
	ampicillin	Polycillin	Labile	Labile
Phenoxy	phenoxymethyl penicillin	Pen-Vee, V-Cillin, Penicillin V, Compocillin	Stable	Labile
	phenethicillin	Darcil, Maxipen, Syncillin	Stable	Labile
Isoxazolyl	oxacillin	Prostaphlin Resistopen	Stable	Stable
	cloxacillin	Tegopen	Stable	Stable
Miscella-neous	methicillin	Staphcillin, Dimocillin	Labile	Stable
	nafcillin	Unipen	Stable	Stable

* Those drugs that are acid-labile should be given primarily by injection or in very high oral dose to be effective. Acid-stable drugs are effective both orally and parenterally. Only the penicillinase-stable drugs are efficacious for the so-called penicillin-resistant staphylococcal infections.

Since all of the penicillins are antigenically related, the patient who is sensitive to one form of penicillin will probably react to any other type. Penicillin sensitivity should be respected, since the anaphylactic penicillin reaction is frequently fatal if not treated promptly. Whenever a penicillin injection is given, a sterile syringe and needle and an ampule of 1:1000 aqueous epinephrine should be available. Although briefly popular, a commercial penicillinase (Neutrapen) is rarely used now for therapy of penicillin reactions. Its onset of activity is too slow to be useful for acute anaphylactic reactions; most other reactions are self-limited, even though troublesome. Since penicillinase is itself a protein enzyme, it may sensitize the patient and do more harm than good.

For the penicillin-sensitive patient, a new drug now available is similar in its general chemical structure and antibacterial spectrum to penicillin, but with a sufficiently small difference in chemical configuration to make it not cross-reactive. Cephalothin (Keflin) can be given to patients with penicillin allergy. It is acid-labile and must be given parenterally. In adults, 0.5 to 1.0 gm every 4 to 6 hours is usually effective against *Pneumococcus, Streptococcus, Staphylococcus* (including penicillin-resistant strains), *E. coli,* some *Aerobacter,* and some *Proteus* species.

Penicillin Substitutes. Before the development of cephalothin and the semisynthetic penicillins, patients who were intolerant of penicillin or had a penicillin-resistant staphylococcal infection required treatment with antibiotics that were totally different. Although this problem is now less compelling, some of these drugs still have a place in clinical therapy.

Erythromycin (Ilosone, Erythrocin, and Ilotycin) is the prototype of a group of antibiotics with large complex molecules called macrolides. Although these antibiotics are effective against all Gram-positive cocci, they should be used primarily for the treatment of staphylococcal infections, although they may also be effective in *Hemophilus* infections and in syphilis. In general, they are usually combined with another antibiotic to prevent or delay the emergence or selection of resistant staphylococci. The usual adult dose is 0.5 gm every 6 hours, orally or intravenously; alternatively 100 mg every 8 to 12 hours may be given deep intramuscularly —deep because it is painful. Side-effects are rare, but intrahepatic cholestasis with jaundice is seen occasionally in patients given erythromycin estolate (Ilosone) for 10 days or longer. The jaundice clears when the drug is discontinued, and no permanent damage has been reported.

Lincomycin (Lincocin) is a new antibiotic of the macrolide type that is very similar to erythromycin. Although organisms that are resistant to lincomycin will be resistant to erythromycin, the converse is not necessarily true, and lincomycin has been used successfully to treat staphylococcal infections that are resistant to both benzyl penicillin and erythromycin. Since it has been introduced so recently, however, there is insufficient experience on which to base any firm opinions with regard to its effectiveness.

The other macrolide antibiotics—oleandomycin (Cyclamycin and Matromycin) triacetyloleandomycin (TAO), spiramycin (Rovamycin), and carbomycin (Magnamycin)—had a brief period of popularity, but have fallen into general disuse because erythromycin is more active than any of them and because resistance to them develops quite easily.

Novobiocin (Albamycin and Cathomycin) is occasionally used in combination with another antibiotic for infections due to staphylococci or to *P. mirabilis* or *P. vulgaris*. It is available for both oral and parenteral use, but a high incidence of skin rashes has limited its use.

Vancomycin (Vancocin) and ristocetin (Spontin) are highly active against Gram-positive cocci, including penicillin-resistant staphylococci. However, they can be administered only intravenously and have a rather high toxicity that limits their use to relatively desperate cases in major medical centers.

Broad-Spectrum Antibiotics. These drugs are active against many Gram-positive and Gram-negative bacteria, some rickettsia, and some of the larger viruses. A large proportion of hospital strains of staphylococci, some streptococci, and occasional strains of pneumococci are resistant. The drugs are bacteriostatic—that is, they halt the growth of bacteria without killing them and rely on the body's natural defenses for elimination of the infection.

CHLORAMPHENICOL.   Chloramphenicol (Chloromycetin) was the first broad-spectrum antibiotic to be isolated and the first antibiotic to be synthesized. The commercial product available today is wholly synthetic. The drug is highly effective; since it is dispensed in tablets, capsules, syrups, drops, or in intramuscular or intravenous preparations, it has become extremely popular. However, one should be very cautious in using chloramphenicol because of its potential toxicity. Although the incidence of bone-marrow depression with pancytopenia (so-called aplastic anemia) is only 1 in 10,000 to 1 in 50,000 cases treated, more than 50 per cent of those who thus develop aplastic anemia die as a direct result. The tragedy is compounded by the fact that most of the fatalities have occured in patients who received the drug for trivial infections. Many of these cases were in the families of physicians, nurses, and pharmacists who treated themselves or their relatives. The use of chloramphenicol should be restricted to the following: (1) typhoid fever or other *Salmonella* infections; (2) *He-*

mophilus influenzae meningitis or tracheobronchitis; (3) meningitis of unknown etiology until the causative organism is identified and more specific therapy initiated; and (4) any serious infection in which there is bacterial or clinical evidence that a less toxic antibiotic cannot be used or where there is convincing evidence that chloramphenicol is the drug of choice for some other reason.

While it is useful to do complete blood counts (including a reticulocyte count) at frequent intervals during the administration of chloramphenicol and to discontinue the drug when the counts fall, this is not always helpful. More often than not, the aplastic anemia develops after the drug has been discontinued. In fact, those cases that show a fall in reticulocyte count, hemoglobin, and hematocrit and a rise in the serum iron (clear signs of toxicity) during the course of chloramphenicol therapy usually recover completely following the cessation of drug therapy. Thus, we cannot emphasize too strongly the fact that, although the risk is small, the consequences of an aplastic anemia caused by chloramphenicol are so dreadful that the drug should be used only on the indications mentioned above.

TETRACYCLINE. The tetracycline group of antibiotics includes chlortetracycline (Aureomycin), oxytetracycline (Terramycin), tetracycline (Achromycin, Tetracyn, Panmycin, Polycycline, Steclin, Sumycin and Tetrex) and demethylchlortetracycline (Declomycin). There is very little difference between any of these in their spectrum of activity or bacterial cross resistance. There are slight differences in absorption; consequently, tetracycline, chlortetracycline, and oxytetracycline are usually given to adults in a dose of 250 to 500 mg every

6 hours, while the comparable dose of demethylchlor-tetracycline is usually 150 mg every 6 hours or 300 mg every 12 hours orally. The parenteral doses are the same for all four drugs: 100 mg every 8 to 12 hours for the intramuscular preparation and 500 mg every 8 to 12 hours by slow drip for the intravenous preparation. With intravenous use, liver toxicity has been reported with daily doses exceeding 1.5 gm, especially in patients with impaired renal function. When outdated drug is used, there is a danger of Fanconi's syndrome, which is usually reversible when the drug is discontinued.

STREPTOMYCIN. The streptomycin group of anti-biotics is usually considered as a separate category of antimicrobials, but streptomycin is really a broad-spectrum antibiotic in some ways. It is effective against some Gram-positive bacteria (it is frequently used in combination with penicillin for this purpose), against most Gram-negative bacteria (in combination with a tetracycline), and against tuberculosis (in combination with isoniazid or para-aminosalicylic acid). Streptomycin should always be used in combination with some other antibiotic because resistance to it develops very rapidly. Streptomycin is given intramuscularly, 0.5 to 1.0 gm every 12 hours, because it is not absorbed from the gastrointestinal tract. The major toxicity is a vestibular disturbance, with vertigo and tinnitus. In elderly persons, with prolonged treatment or high dosage there also may be deafness and renal toxicity. The incidence of deafness was so high with dihydrostreptomycin that it was removed from the market. In general, streptomycin should not be used for more than 7 to 10 days, except in the therapy of tuberculosis. The other members of the streptomycin group—kanamycin sulfate

(Kantrex), paromomycin sulfate (Humatin), and neomycin (many trade names)—are rarely used for systemic
therapy because of a high incidence of renal and oto-
toxicity. They are used mainly in topical perparations;
because they are so poorly absorbed, they are frequently
given prior to surgery to reduce the bacterial flora of
the gastrointestinal tract.

Polypeptide Antibiotics. These drugs are relatively
simple chemicals, but they have a moderately high toxicity that limits their systemic use to very special situations. However, they have been used extensively in
topical preparations for the skin, ear, and eye. Bacitra-
cin (many trade names), polymyxin B (Aerosporin), and
tyrothricin (Tyotocin) are the most popular and are
often compounded with neomycin. Occasionally, polymyxin B or colistin (Coly-Mycin) is used systemically (intramuscularly) for the treatment of a *Pseudomonas* or
Proteus infection that is resistant to other antibiotics.
In such cases, one must watch for renal and neurological toxicity and use these drugs with full knowledge of
how the anticipated therapeutic ends will balance
against the predictable toxicity. In a life-threatening
septicemia, almost any risk is justified.

SULFONAMIDES

The antibacterial activity of the dye prontosil was
discovered in 1932 and the active component, sulfanil-
amide, was isolated in 1936. Since then, many thousands
of sulfonamides with modifications of structure have
been synthesized by chemists. Some of these are more
and some less soluble, some more easily inactivated or
longer lasting, and some have even found uses unrelat-

ed to antibacterial effects. At present, sulfonamides are used chiefly for urinary-tract infections caused mainly by *E. coli*. They are also used in meningococcal and nocardial infections, for *H. influenzae* infections (supplementary to antibiotics), in bacillary dysentery, toxoplasmosis, glanders, meliodosis, lymphogranuloma venereum, chanchroid, and some gastrointestinal inflammations.

The mechanism of action of sulfonamides is of great interest and points the way to methods of synthesizing more effective drugs. Both animals and bacteria require folic acid for a variety of essential life functions. Animals obtain folic acid from the environment (mostly dietary), whereas many bacteria are so fastidious that they will not accept folic acid from the environment, using only that which they synthesize themselves from para-aminobenzoic acid. Sulfonamides closely resemble this compound and prevent its utilization by the bacteria, which then starve for folic acid while living in an environment with otherwise available folic acid. Animals are not harmed because they do not depend upon para-aminobenzoic acid for their folic acid. The soluble sulfonamides, succinylsulfathiazole (Sulfasuxidine) and phthalylsulfathiazole (Sulfathalidine) are used before abdominal surgery to reduce the bacterial flora of the intestinal tract.

A variety of preparations is available for urinary-tract infections. Sulfadiazine has always been the standard to which newer drugs are compared. It is usually given to adults in a dose of 1.0 gm every 6 hours following a loading dose of 2 to 4 gm. The objection to this drug is that a good urinary output must be maintained; otherwise, there is a danger that crystals of the drug will form in the kidneys. Alkalinization of the urine helps to avoid this. The use of triple sulfa preparations is based on the fact that the solubility of each sulfa compound is independent of the others used simultaneously. Thus, the same total dose of three sulfonamides (usually sulfadiazine, sulfamerazine, and sulfamethazine) would lead to one-third as much of each drug in the urine; presumably, the solubility of each would then be sufficient to prevent crystalluria. Most investigators believe that this has worked as predicted, but a few are skeptical.

Several sulfonamides have been developed with increased solubility to avoid problems of crystalluria. Some of these, such as sulfisoxazole (Gantrisin), sulfisomidine (Elkosin), and sulfamethizole (Thiosulfil), have achieved great popularity, although there is no convincing evidence that they are any better or safer than sulfadiazine or triple sulfas. In general, they prosper in proportion to local preferences or persuasive advertising.

Several long-acting sulfonamides now available may be dispensed in doses as low as 0.5 gm per day. Aside from the convenience and low cost of taking only one tablet a day, these preparations offer no advantages and may present a disadvantage in the event of a reaction. Such preparations as lipid suspensions of sulfonamides and sulfathidole (Sul-Spansion) may be given every 12 hours. Sulfamethoxypyridazine (Kynex and Midicel) and sulfadimethoxine (Madribon) are usually given 0.5 gm a day in a single dose following a loading dose of 1.0 gm. When using sulfonamides, one should be wary of allergic reactions, hepatic or bone-marrow toxicity, methemoglobinemia, neurological or psychiatric sequelae, and connective-tissue diseases.

URINARY ANTISEPTICS

These agents are neither antibiotics nor sulfonamides, but are concentrated by the kidneys into the urine, where they destroy bacteria. Nitrofurantoin (Furadantin) is useful for the treatment of urinary-tract infection caused by *Proteus, E. coli,* and some *Staphylococcus* and less often those caused by *Aerobacter* and *Streptococcus*. It is usually given orally to adults in a dose of 50 to 100 mg every 6 hours. An intravenous preparation is also available for very special situations. Nausea, vomiting, and rashes frequently accompany therapy; in patients with a hereditary deficiency of the enzyme glucose-6-phosphate dehydrogenase in their red blood cells, hemolytic anemias commonly occur.

Methenamine mandelate (Mandelamine) is a combination of methenamine and mandelic acid. The methenamine is a condensation product of formaldehyde and ammonia. When the urine is acidic, formaldehyde is liberated from the methenamine and exerts a bactericidal effect locally. The mandelic acid is excreted unchanged and also exerts a bactericidal effect in acid urine. The usual adult dose is 1.0 gm every 6 to 8 hours; special measures may be required to keep the urine acid in the range of pH 5.5 to 6.0.

COMMON CAUSES OF FAILURE OF ANTIBACTERIAL THERAPY

A great many factors can lead to failure of the therapeutic effect, but some are extremely common. For example, an incorrect diagnosis of a sore throat caused by a virus and not a bacterium will doom any antibiotic therapy to failure. A lesion that is inaccessible to the drug—an abscess or undebrided necrotic tissue, for example—will not respond. Neither will an infection that is treated by the improper drug or by the correct drug given by an ineffective route, in an insufficient dosage or for too short a period of time. Patients with impaired host defenses—those with a malignancy or on steroid therapy or antineoplastic immunosuppressive drugs—will generally fail to respond to bacteriostatic agents and require unusually large doses of bactericidal agents. If the infecting bacterium is resistant to the drug or a resistant population is selected by the drug, then therapy is not likely to succeed unless a new drug or combination of drugs to which the infecting agent is sensitive is used. Finally, inappropriate attempts at antibacterial prophylaxis are usually doomed to failure. When broad-spectrum antibiotics are used to treat the possible bacterial complications of a simple self-limited viral disease, superinfection with resistant organisms frequently results. It is best to treat bacterial infections as they arise except in the case of penicillin prophylaxis against streptococci in patients with rheumatic fever.

HAZARDS OF ANTIBACTERIAL THERAPY

In addition to the multitude of benefits that have resulted from the antibacterial drugs, a great many hazards also occur. Many allergic phenomena, ranging from anaphylaxis with fatalities to serum sickness and skin rashes are seen. Some drugs cause bone-marrow aplasia, agranulocytosis, hepatitis, nausea, vomiting, diarrhea, vertigo, or deafness. Antibacterial agents sometimes mask serious disease when given indiscriminately, and appendicitis or mastoiditis may escape detection. Careless use of antibiotics can lead to superinfection with drug-resistant organisms in the individual, and may even foster the development of resistant strains in the community. Unnecessary antibiotics also represent a heavy expense to patients.

Sedatives, Hypnotics, and Tranquilizers

A variety of drugs act on the central nervous system; these include many drugs with overlapping qualities. For clarity, it is best to define our terms despite some duplication. *Sedatives* are drugs used to calm a patient without causing sleep. *Hypnotics* are drugs used to put patients to sleep; many hypnotics are used in reduced dosage as sedatives. *Tranquilizers* are more difficult to define. The term was devised as an advertising phrase rather than as a descriptive scientific name. A tranquilizer is now generally defined as a drug that calms and sedates without causing hypnosis or anesthesia.

SEDATIVES AND HYPNOTICS

The first sedative-hypnotic to be used was the bromide ion. It has no place in modern medicine. Perhaps the safest and best hypnotic-sedative is chloral hydrate. It is used in hard gelatin capsules or tablets and has a wide margin of safety. For sedation, 0.25 gm is usually sufficient; for sleep, 0.5 to 1.0 gm may be used. This is the agent of choice for the elderly patient. Chloral betaine (Beta-Chlor) is a combination of chloral hydrate and betaine. Its action is identical to that of chloral hydrate, but with virtual elimination of undesirable gastrointestinal effects. The hypnotic dose is 870 to 1700 mg at bedtime. It must be used with extreme caution (if at all) in patients with liver or renal disease.

Barbiturates are the most popular hynotic-sedatives, but in the very young or in the elderly person they may cause excitement rather than the anticipated effect. Therefore, barbiturates must be used cautiously at the extremes of age. Phenobarbital (Luminal), pentobarbital (Nembutal), secobarbital (Seconal), and butabarbital (Butisol) are all generally used in an adult dose of 100 mg for hypnosis, but a lesser dose is advised for the elderly person if barbiturates are to be used at all.

Many nonbarbiturate hypnotic-sedatives are available, but they offer no particular advantage over those already mentioned except as personal preferences based on individual experience. Such agents and their usual adult dosages are listed in Table 2, but lower doses should be used in the elderly.

TABLE 2

Nonbarbiturate hypnotic-sedatives

Generic Name	Trade Name	Usual Bedtime Adult Hypnotic Dose
ethchlorvynol	Placidyl	0.5 to 1.0 gm
ethinamate	Valmid	1.0 gm
oxanamide	Quiactin	0.8 gm
methprylon	Noludar	0.2 to 0.4 gm
glutethimide	Doriden	0.5 to 1.0 gm
ectylurea	Nostyn	300 to 600 mg
methylparafynol	Dormison	250 to 750 mg

NOTE: For the elderly the above "usual" doses are probably too high, and a lower dose should be tried first.

Many physicians prefer to use antihistamines for sedation in the elderly and pediatric age groups. For adults, diphenhydramine (Benadryl), o.1 gm, or promethazine (Phenergan), 25 mg, are recommended. They are safe and usually effective.

TRANQUILIZERS

Tranquilizers are usually classified as minor, intermediate, and major. The minor tranquilizers are very similar to sedatives.

Recently, meprobamate (Miltown and Equanil) was reclassified by the U.S. Pharmacopeia Committee as a hypnotic-sedative, although it had been regarded as a tranquilizer for many years and was perhaps the most widely used of that group. It is also a weak muscle relaxant. A similar drug is phenaglycodol (Ultran). These are mild, safe agents, but can cause coma and death with massive overdosage. The usual meprobamate dose is 200 to 400 mg 3 times a day; 1600 mg is an absolutely maximal adult dose. The usual adult dose of phenaglycodol is also 200 to 400 mg 3 times daily.

Two mild tranquilizers were originally developed as antihistaminics. Benzactyzine (Suavitil and Phobex) and hydroxyzine (Atarax and Vistaril) appear to be useful and safe tranquilizers for all age groups. Hydroxyzine is also useful as an antiemetic and has been reported to protect the heart against epinephrine-induced arrhythmias.

At present, the most popular and widely used mild tranquilizer is chlordiazepoxide (Librium). It has some muscle-relaxant properties and is a mild euphoriant. Some success has been reported with this drug in the treatment of alcoholic patients with delirium tremens.

Although it is related to meprobamate in activity, it is more potent and broader in scope. The usual dosage for geriatric patients is 5 mg 2 to 4 times a day. Young adults tolerate higher dosages.

The major tranquilizers are used for patients with severe emotional problems. These are potent drugs and have revolutionized the situation in mental hospitals by making the patients more manageable so that psychotherapy may become possible. However, the potency of these drugs also increases their potential toxicity. In general, these drugs fall into two major groups: (1) the *Rauwolfia* alkaloids, and (2) the phenothiazine derivatives.

The *Rauwolfia* alkaloids are derived from an Indian snakeroot. They were introduced originally for the treatment of hypertension. By the oral route, the onset of drug action follows a latent period of several days; when a parenteral route is employed, drug effects may be noted in a few hours. When used as psychotherapeutic agents, the *Rauwolfia* alkaloids produce a peaceful state so that the patient does not react with very much emotion to situations about him. Patients relax better, go to sleep more readily, but perform normally. This group of drugs is good for the control of agitated, tense, and anxious individuals with psychoneurotic behavior. Mild untoward effects are common and include diarrhea, nasal obstruction, and an increase in appetite. Less common but more dangerous complications that have been noted include: (1) increased gastric acidity and motility, often leading to peptic ulcer with hemorrhage; (2) mental depression, occasionally leading to suicide; (3) extrapyramidal effects, the clinical picture of parkinsonism with a pill-rolling tremor with some rigidity; (4) fluid retention, occasionally leading to congestive heart failure; and (5) vascular collapse during surgery. Since these untoward effects are more common in the elderly patient, this group of drugs must be used with extreme caution. The members of the *Rauwolfia* group and their common dosages are listed in Table 3.

TABLE 3

Rauwolfia drugs

Generic Name	Trade Name	Usual Adult Dosage	Composition
reserpine	Serpasil, Sandril	0.1 to 0.25 mg per day	Purified alkaloid
rescinnamine	Moderil	0.25 to 0.5 mg twice per day	Purified alkaloid
deserpidine	Harmonyl	0.1 to 0.25 mg per day	Purified alkaloid
alseroxylon	Rauwiloid	1 to 2 tablets per day	Alkaloid mixture
rauwolfia serpentina	Raudixin	100 to 200 mg per day	Crude root
syrosingopine	Singoserp	1 to 2 mg per day	Synthetic analogue

The phenothiazine derivatives have been used extensively to relieve agitation in the aged and the senile and to reduce delusions, hallucinations, and disorderly behavior. They sedate the patient without causing clouding of the mental processes or confusion. There is some evidence that confused and memory-impaired patients function better with these drugs because they remove emotional interference and suppress agitation, excitement, tension, psychoneurotic anxiety, and fear. In addition, these drugs are antiemetic and antipruritic, and they potentiate and prolong the action of sedatives, hypnotics, narcotics, and anesthetics.

Most experience with phenothiazines in the treatment of psychoses has been accumulated using chlorpromazine (Thorazine) in doses ranging from 10 to 1000 mg per day. Doses higher than 25 mg should not be used except by physicians having considerable experience in psychotherapeutics. High doses tend to increase the incidence of such untoward effects as orthostatic hypotension, disturbed heat regulation, skin rashes, extrapyramidal symptoms, and increased appetite.

The basic phenothiazine molecule has been used to develop a large number of derivatives with different properties. Some are long-acting, with great potency, but are more prone to produce extrapyramidal symptoms. Some are better as antiemetics and some as antipruritics; some are more sedative, while others tend to be alerting. The better antiemetics include prochlorperazine (Compazine), perphenazine (Trilafon), thioperazine (Vontil), thiethylperazine (Torecan), trimethobenzamide (Tigan), and trifluoperazine (Stelazine). The best antipruritics are trimeprazine (Temaril) and methdilazine (Tacaryl). Trifluoperazine (Stelazine) has been used extensively in the elderly patient because of its alerting properties. However, physicians tend to have their individual favorite drugs; as they gain experience with any particular derivative, they tend to use it more effectively so that, in their hands, this turns out to be the best drug for their patients. A partial list of phenothiazone tranquilizers is included below without dosages because these tend to vary with the therapeutic indication.

TABLE 4

Phenothiazine Tranquilizers

Generic Name	Trade Name
chlorpromazine	Thorazine, Largactil
promazine	Sparine
triflupromazine	Vesprin
methoxypromazine	Tentone
promethazine	Phenergan
thioridazine	Mellaril
trimeprazine	Temaril
ethopropazine	Parsidol
prochlorperazine	Compazine
trifluoperazine	Stelazine
thioperazine	Vontil
thiethylperazine	Torecan
perphenazine	Trilafon
fluphenazine	Prolixin, Permitil
acetophenazine	Tindal
thiopropazate	Dartal
pipamazine	Mornidine
methdilazine	Tacaryl
mepazine	Pacatal
trimethobenzamide	Tigan

When extrapyramidal symptoms develop during phenothiazine therapy, treatment should be with such anti-parkinsonian drugs as diphenhydramine (Benadryl), benztropine (Congentin), or trihexyphenidyl (Artane), or some combination of these.

Antihypertensive Drugs

Hypertension may have any one of several causes. In each case, the best therapy is to remove or prevent the underlying cause—for example, unilateral renal disease, pheochromocytoma, chronic pyelonephritis, acute glomerulonephritis, and arteriolar nephrosclerosis. However, 95 per cent of all cases of hypertension are idiopathic, that is, no cause is known, although there seems to be some association with stress. In the absence of an understanding of etiology, therapy must be empiric; this usually implies trial and error.

The earliest effective agents used in the treatment of hypertension were the sedatives. These are still an important aspect of therapy, although they passed into temporary eclipse when the *Rauwolfia* drugs became popular. The *Rauwolfia* alkaloids are still used extensively, especially for the milder cases, but their toxicity is potentially great.

For the severe cases of hypertension, attempts were made to block the sympathetic nervous system peripherally with a variety of ganglionic blocking agents. These drugs have evolved from the relatively non-specific and highly toxic hexamethonium (Bistrium) through pentolinium (Ansolysen) and mecamylamine (Inversine), to bretylium tosylate (Darenthin) and guanethidine (Ismelin), which are safer, more dependable, and more potent. At the moment, guanethidine is the most popular blocking agent. Although the usual beginning dosage is 10 mg per day, the drug must be titrated to the requirements of the individual patient.

Hydralazine (Apresoline) is a unique drug that acts both centrally and peripherally to reduce blood pressure; it dilates the renal blood vessels and increases renal blood flow. At one time, this drug was widely used, and good results were reported, especially when it was combined with a ganglionic blocking agent. Prolonged use led to a significant number of cases of "hydralazine syndrome," a drug-induced illness very similar to systemic lupus erythematosus, which usually remitted after cessation of drug administration. Although it is safe when used carefully, hydralazine is no longer widely used.

Diuretics have been found to reduce blood pressure after several days of administration as total body sodium becomes depleted. The earliest experience was accumulated with chlorothiazide (Diuril), about 0.5 gm per day. Many experts now place all their hypertensives on some oral diuretic, usually of the thiazide type, and then build with other drugs on this foundation if the response is unsatisfactory with the diuretic alone. There are now several dozen thiazide diuretics that can be used for this purpose. Restriction of salt or sodium intake alone will often give comparable results.

In previous years, such inhibitors of the central sympathetic function as the veratrum alkaloids, the proto-veratrines A and B, were used to reduce blood pressure. Although almost invariably effective, the therapeutic dose was so close to the dose that caused severe nausea and vomiting that the drug was usually unacceptable to patients and has now fallen into disuse.

Recently, the aldosterone antagonist, spironolactone (Aldactone-A), has been used to increase sodium excretion by opposing the actions of aldosterone. It does not promote potassium excretion; since its action is weak when used alone, it has been used in combination with the thiazides.

In evaluating the therapy of hypertension, there has been considerable controversy over the question of effectiveness. A minority of experts feel that drug therapy neither prolongs life nor reduces morbidity, but only serves to reassure the patient and allow the doctor to feel that he is "doing something." The great majority of experts point out that in the case of malignant hypertension, where life expectancy is predictably very short, drug therapy has led to a very marked prolongation of life and a major reduction in morbidity. In mild cases of hypertension, there is no convincing evidence that drug therapy has a comparable efficacy, but most physicians believe that such a relationship will become evident with more experience and better techniques of evaluation. In any case, therapy seems indicated so long as it is safe and effective without causing toxicity.

Laxatives

Constipation is a common complaint of many elderly people. To treat this symptom successfully, one should fully understand the normal physiology of the intestinal tract. There can be considerable variation in what is considered "normal." Cases are on record of normal patients who have had no bowel movement for many weeks and yet have had no dysfunction. It is generally accepted that the normal function consists of bowel movements that occur daily or within a period of several days. The ingestion of food material is followed by peristalsis in the intestinal tract. Segmentation also assists in these involuntary muscular movements. Defecation follows other reflex stimulation from the nerves of the large bowel. The fecal material is composed of water, mucus, bile, mineral salts, and unabsorbed food particles. The last is commonly referred to as roughage. The restriction of physical activity and of the amounts of food and water ingested tends to reduce the amount of fecal material discharged.

One should not overlook the fact that fecal impaction or intestinal obstruction from tumors can be the cause of increasing constipation: diverticulitis, mucous colitis, and other diseases must be considered. Enemas of plain water, or retention enemas of warm mineral oil followed by a plain water enema are sometimes necessary to free fecal impactions. Corrective steps should then be taken to change any poor habits. These are also determined by the patient's physical condition. If the patient's general condition warrants, he should be encouraged to do mild physical exercise. Adequate amounts of fluid and fruit juices are recommended; prune juice is helpful. Whole fruit is preferred to fruit juice. Spinach, lettuce, and other green vegetables help to provide bulk in nonabsorbed material. These measures should be checked for each patient.

If drugs are required, the mild laxatives should be tried first. Bulk can be provided with agar, psyllium, methyl cellulose, carol gum, and bran. Mineral oil has long been used. Some authorities claim that liquid petrolatum prevents the absorption of vitamins and that it can cause other pathological changes, although such changes have not been clearly proved. Cascara sagrada is a mild and reliable laxative. Aloe and calomel are not recommended. Phenolphthalein, which acts briefly and effectively on the intestinal tract can sometimes cause skin rashes. The saline cathartics, such as magnesium sulfate, magnesium citrate, and milk of magnesia act by retaining water in the intestinal tract.

Thus, in the treatment of the constipation, one must first ensure sufficient physical activity and an adequate intake of fluids and bulk materials. If drugs are necessary, the mild laxative should be tried first. Cascara, mixtures of mineral oil and milk of magnesia, or agar, mineral oil, and phenolphthalein are suggested. The rationale of treatment is to return the patient to normal bowel habits.

Decubitus Ulcer

Decubitus ulcers occur in the elderly, undernourished, bedridden patient. The treatment and healing of such ulcers requires good nursing care and attention. The patient should have an adequate intake of nutritious food and vitamins. Pressure points should be protected by the use of "doughnuts," lamb's wool, or frequent position changes. Patients' pajamas or nightgowns should be washed in mild soaps; commercial soaps used in the laundering of sheets are found to be irritating to the skin. Strict cleanliness should be observed; poor aseptic techniques by staff and personnel can supply the offending organism that causes an ulcer. Many ointments have been suggested, but adequate nutrition, cleanliness, care of pressure points, and prevention of skin irritation remain the most effective measures in the treatment of this condition.

8

Bacteriology of the Environment

———◆•◆———

THE problem presented by infections acquired by patients in hospitals and nursing homes continues to require attention to improve methods of control. A recent survey in a large Boston hospital showed that the percentage of patients with hospital-acquired infection had risen from 9 per cent in 1956 to 13 per cent in 1964, indicating a gradual upward trend. This parallels the experience of all hospitals that have investigated the problem and demonstrates the extent of cross infection in large institutions providing medical care. Connecticut hospitals have had similar experiences and are confronted from time to time with cross infection. While the usual source is a wound infection, the respiratory tract, the skin, and the genitourinary tract may all be implicated in precipitating an outbreak. *Staphyloccus aureus* is the most frequent offender, followed by the Gram-negative organisms: *Escherichia coli, Proteus* genus, *Klebsiella aerobacter,* and *Pseudomonas aeruginosa.*

The concern of the nurse and the physician in the nursing home is to familiarize themselves with the insidious cycle of infection starting with the infected patient, the reservoirs of bacteria created in the nursing-home enviroment, the disseminating carriers among nursing-home personnel, and the means of transmission among these three epidemiological components. The patient may have an abscess of the skin, an infection in his nose and throat, or an infection in the kidney or bowel. Whatever the site of the infection, this patient is a shedder of bacteria into the enviroment: the air in the room, the bed linen, and the floor. Although the skin abscess is covered by a clean dressing, bacteria will filter through it and be found about the adjacent skin areas. The urine and excreta from the infected patient also serve to contaminate the clothing and bed linen. We are aware of the spread of microorganisms by direct contact from person to person, but we are less aware of their spread by other means.

Dissemination of Bacteria

The fact that air currents transport bacteria was established by Carl Flugge in 1897. His work was not considered significant and was forgotten until 1936, when W. F. Wells pointed out that bacteria were disseminated in three ways: by droplets, by droplet nuclei, and by dust. Droplets are defined as particles larger than 100 microns in size; dust particles vary from 10 to 100 microns in size; and droplet nuclei range from 2 to 10 microns in size. When discharged by coughing and sneezing, droplets settle to the floor rapidly. The dust particles which arise from lint, particles of feathers, wool, or skin are suspended in the air and settle out more slowly. The droplet nuclei are much more likely to float about in the air currents until they are inhaled or removed by ventilation; they constitute the greatest hygienic hazard for respiratory-tract infection. Riley and Wells actually demonstrated that air from patients with active tuberculosis could infect guinea pigs and thereby proved that air is an important factor in the spread of pulmonary disease.

The density of bacteria in the air and the fallout rate depends on the presence of shedders, bacterial contamination, location, air currents, movement of personnel, and humidity. Studies have shown, for example, that the fallout rate in a laundry-sorting area can be 300 bacteria per square foot per minute, whereas in a clean operating room the rate is 2 to 5 bacteria. In a patient's room during bedmaking, the fallout is 50 to 260 bacteria; during no activity it is 15 to 50 bacteria.

ENVIRONMENTAL RESERVOIRS

Next to the patient himself, his pillowcases, sheets, and blankets have the highest concentration of bacteria. A pillowcase can harbor 68,000 organisms per square foot, and a top sheet 38,000 organisms: however, the underside of the top sheet on culture will show less than 500 organisms. The patient's clothing is also covered with bacteria. The fallout from the air of these bacteria particles lands on horizontal surfaces. Thus the floor of the room, as the largest horizontal surface, is a large reservoir of septic debris. Table tops, dresser tops, and all horizontal ledges are contaminated as well. Other reservoirs of bacteria are carpets, ice ma-

chines, bedside carafes, air conditioners, and inhalation
equipment; these are discussed below under the head-
ing Control of Cross Infection. Movement in the
room, bed changing, and other factors that create air
currents tend to return bacteria particles from the environmental reservoirs to suspension in the air.

CARRIERS

Not all patients with pathogenic bacteria become
infected. Tests on healthy, healing surgical wounds have
shown bacteria to be present. Wound healing depends
on the dosage of bacteria, the virulence of the organism,
and the patient's immunity. The infected patient usually
becomes a carrier; as such, he transmits bacteria to
others and to his environment from two sources: the
lesion as well as the nasopharynx.

The personnel in a hospital or nursing home may become carriers from contact with the infected patient
and his environment, or from contact with ill members
of their families at home. Outer clothing of the personnel becomes contaminated by caring for the infected
patient. Such clothing can increase the bacteria of the
air to a count of 700 per cubic foot. One can visualize
the possibilities of spread when an attendant changes
bed linen, disseminating many organisms about her—
on her clothing and into the environment.

The nasopharnyx is the most frequent site of colonization of organisms in carriers, although such other
sites as skin, groin, and perineum have been reported.
Once an area is colonized, it remains an excellent and
frequently a persistent reservoir. One has only to observe a person who exhales when smoking to observe
the pattern and spread of exhaled air. Investigations

have shown that persons sitting in an open ward of patients can become colonized after four hours of exposure to the air. Furthermore, the organisms with which they become colonized are the organisms predominating in the ward. In one study, for example, nasal cultures of student nurses at the beginning of training showed that 29 per cent were carriers of antibiotic-resistant S. aureus: after 18 months in a hospital, 87 per cent were carrying this germ, an increase of almost 60 per cent. In another example of carrier dissemination, a laboratory technician standing on the periphery of an operating room was able to infect two patients. He had an unusual phage type that was positively identified as the causative organism. The laboratory coat of this carrier was studied with an air centrifuge; 160 S. aureus of his phage type were recovered in 5 cubic feet, and the fallout per square foot per minute was 44 organisms.

Carrier studies were made in one hospital that was experiencing a high incidence of S. aureus phage Type 80/81. The distribution of carriers was found to be widespread throughout the hospital staff. Two surgeons were carriers: one of them had been treating a chronic osteomyelitis with phage Type 80/81 for months. An operating-room nurse, the operating orderly, several nurses on the patient floors, personnel in housekeeping, and the dietary personnel were all carriers of the organism. When such organisms are present, obviously the carriers can be found in all departments and all hospital areas—the hospital has become a reservoir. This same type of carrier dissemination can occur in the nursing home.

Some simple tests can be carried out to observe and

study enviromental contamination. If air-sampling devices are not available, blood agar Petri dishes exposed to the air will accumulate fallout from the airborne suspension. The nursing home can then send the Petri dishes to an outside laboratory for cultural tests and reports. It has been found, for example, that such a Petri dish placed on an operating table or delivery table after the room has been cleaned, and with no activity, will have a fallout of 1 to 3 colonies per square foot per minute, whereas another such dish exposed in the laundry-sorting area will have 120 colonies or more in the same period of time. One can test linen and textiles by impression plates. This method consists of taking a clean glass, inverting it, wiping the flat bottom with alcohol, placing the cloth over it, and pressing it against a Petri dish. Nose and throat cultures can be obtained more easily by having the patient wear a mask over the nose and mouth and then imprinting the face side of the mask on the agar plate.

Control of Cross Infection

Methods of control must be instituted immediately whenever an increase in the infection rate in a facility caring for patients is recognized. The patient who is infected and is a shedder must be isolated. Isolation techniques already being practiced must be reevaluated.

LOCATION OF WORK AREAS

Utility areas must be completely separated into clean and soiled work areas. One cannot be expected to maintain satisfactory techniques when sterile medications are prepared adjacent to soiled material.

Handling of Linens. The handling of linens requires careful attention. As has been previously pointed out, the pillows, sheets, and blankets are grossly contaminated. When the bed is changed, care should be used to remove the soiled linen with a minimum of motion, and it should be placed in a hamper on a moveable stand. The soiled linen should be covered when transported. Carrying soiled linen loosely to the laundry chute or packing it into soiled pillowcases contaminates the attendant and disseminates clouds of dust particles throughout the area. Linen from infected patients should be bagged, identified, and handled separately. Laundry procedures should include the use of hot water (180°F.) and a bactericidal agent in the final rinse to ensure destruction of organisms.

RECOMMENDATIONS FOR CLEANING

The horizontal areas of the environment are the greatest reservoirs of bacteria. Staphylococci mixed with blood, pus, or amniotic fluid will survive for 24 hours; on a clean dry surface they will die within 8 hours. *P. aeruginosa* has been found to persist for 2 months in wards where burn patients were cared for. These pathogens must therefore be destroyed by germicidal detergents. Although dry-mopping a floor may remove gross debris, tests have shown that mopping spreads bacteria through the environment. Wet mopping also has many disadvantages; unless mop heads and water containing germicidal detergents are frequently changed, they spread organisms from one room to another and actually paint all floors with a thin layer of bacteria. Wet vacuuming has become the method of choice. It is possible to maintain operating-room floors at 5 organisms per square centimeter and a patient's room floor at 10 organisms per square centimeter by using germicidal detergents and flooding the floor. The solution must be left on the surface for from 5 to 10 minutes to be bactericidal. Synthetic phenolics, quaternaries, and iodophors are all agents that may be used. A quart of solution made up according to the manufacturer's directions is poured on the floor and mopped with a clean mop to loosen debris. Several quarts of additional solution are then spread with the mop and allowed to remain on the floor. The solution is removed with a wet pickup vacuum cleaner. Daily cleaning of critical areas such as the infected patient's room (and all adjacent areas during an outbreak of infection) is recommended. Routine cleaning of patient areas once a week by this method is adequate under normal conditions.

It is recommended that dry vacuuming be the method used in the interval between wet vacuuming. Many vacuum cleaners are equipped with filters that will prevent the dissemination of bacteria. Floor waxes with an added germicide are recommended, since it has been found that waxes without this additive may be contaminated with Gram-negative organisms. Written procedures for floor care are necessary if schedules are to be carried out as planned and if housekeeping is to be scientific and not haphazard.

In summary, the following cleaning procedures are recommended:

1. Work teams should be trained to clean patient-care areas.
2. Properly designed wet and dry vacuum cleaners must be supplied.

3. Informed supervision is essential to enforce proper use of germicidal detergents and maintenance of machines. A good germicide falls in one of the three following categories: iodophor, synthetic phenolic, or quaternary.
4. Cleaning time must be scheduled and regarded as an integral part of patient care.
5. Floors should be disinfected by wet pickup technique weekly, except in such critical areas as operating rooms, utility rooms, and isolation rooms, where daily disinfection should be carried out.
6. Furniture should be dusted with cloths dampened with a germicidal detergent.
7. Vacuum cleaners must be used in place of mops, brushes, and brooms in daily care of floors between periodic disinfection by a wet pickup technique.
8. Trash and linen should be collected in a manner designed to prevent dispersal of bacteria.

CONTROL OF OTHER ENVIRONMENTAL RESERVOIRS

Carpets have no place in patient-care areas. They are unsanitary and rapidly become stained and contaminated. Moreover, they constitute an unnecessary fire hazard.

Ice-making and ice-storage machines are frequent reservoirs of bacteria. The cold and moisture favor the prolonged survival of bacteria. The ice scoop with its handle, as well as the human hand, introduce organisms into the ice-storage compartment.

Bedside carafes have been found contaminated with patient's organisms. Patients drinking from them with straws deposit their bacteria therein through reflux of saliva. They are also contaminated through handling by attendants. Many carafes are made with small-mouthed openings that prevent easy cleaning and also made from materials that cannot withstand the 170° F. temperature required for sanitizing dishes. No matter what type of carafes are used, they must be identified for each patient so that there can be no interchange. They should have wide-mouthed openings and be constructed of materials to withstand the sanitizing temperature.

The air-conditioner that recirculates air allows bacteria to accumulate in it. The moisture that is present in air-conditioners provides a protected site where bacteria live and grow. When filters are not changed, they become contaminated. Schedules for cleaning of air-conditioners and filters must be planned at regular intervals to prevent them from becoming a source of contamination.

Oxygen-therapy equipment presents problems in cleaning. Studies have shown that simple rinsing of masks is not sufficient to remove the bacteria accumulated during use. Ethylene oxide gas sterilization is the ideal method of caring for such equipment. If this device is not available, one must turn to other means. Equipment can be washed by submerging and scrubbing in a solution of either 75 parts per million of iodophor or a 2 per cent solution of synthetic phenolic, followed by a thorough rinsing in tap water. One can only speculate as to the number of patients who have acquired respiratory infection from contaminated inhalation-therapy equipment that has been improperly cleaned.

The following procedures are recommended for the care of inhalation-therapy equipment:

1. Terminal disinfection of all inhalation therapy equipment with an iodophor with 75 p.p.m. available iodine or a 2 per cent solution of synthetic phenolic is obligatory. The equipment is submerged and thoroughly scrubbed after a minimum contact time of 15 minutes. It is then rinsed thoroughly in tap water.
2. Under no circumstances should plain soap or detergent and water be used in washing contaminated equipment, as bacteria and viruses are not destroyed, and the equipment may come out of the wash water with alkali earth films (soap curd) to trap the bacteria. This practice constitutes a hazard to personnel responsible for the cleaning through splashing of virus- and bacteria-laden water.
3. After cleaning, as indicated in 1 and 2, the equipment may be sterilized by autoclaving if it is constructed of heat-resistant materials. If not, ethylene oxide sterilization is recommended.
4. Humidifiers are presented sterile to each patient. Sterile, distilled water is added at the bedside. One humidifier should never be used for a patient for longer than one week.

The patient's attendant must be constantly aware of the environment in which she is working and the methods for the control of bacterial transmission. Hand-washing facilities with foot-operated soap dispensers should be readily accessible in all areas. A foot-dispensed hand solution is suggested for use between patients where sinks are not available or as an additional precaution following handwashing. Such a solution can be made up in a pharmacy and consists of:

Banzalkomium chloride	10.0 ml
Cetyl alcohol	5.0 gm
Isopropanol or ethanol	665.0 ml
Water q.s.	1000.0 ml

Masks lose 60 per cent of their effectiveness after 20 minutes. When one must be masked continually, the mask should be changed at frequent intervals. The mask prevents some spread of organisms and can be of some protection against colonization. The attendant should change clothing as indicated in both clean and contaminated areas. The attendant must exercise care not to become a carrier.

9
Nutrition

———◆◆———

G o o d nutrition plays a vital role throughout life. Everyone requires certain basic foods that will supply energy and the nutrients required for optimum health. Nursing homes, which are engaged in serving mainly the geriatric patient, are faced with a real challenge in that all the problems of any institutional food program exist in addition to a few that are specific for this age group.

Nursing homes, although varying from the very small to the large institution with several hundred patients, all have the same basic nutritional problems; to a large degree, the same basic principles of operations apply to both types. The successful operation of a dietary service calls for both a nutritional and an administrative approach. The former includes menu planning, with proper emphasis on nutritional content, appetite appeal, and special therapeutic diets; preparation of standardized recipes; supervision of food preparation with reference to proper procedures and sanitary controls; kitchen test to maintain quality of foods, supervision of food service and patient feeding; and training and supervision of personnel. The administrative aspects include such items as purchasing food and supplies, establishing cost controls and accounting, and employing and overseeing personnel, including dietician, cooks, and kitchen and serving personnel.

Nutritional Aspects

The health and contentment of nursing-home patients are greatly influenced by what, where, and how they eat. It is appreciated that meals that have been well planned and attractively prepared are oftentimes as important as good nursing or medical care. Obviously, administrators of nursing homes and the dietician have a responsibility to provide the kind of food services that will meet these needs. As mentioned above, nursing-home patients present certain additional nutritional problems that must be considered before a food program can be set up.

SPECIAL PROBLEMS AFFECTING THE AGED

Patients often arrive at the nursing home in various stages of physical debility and malnutrition, which must be corrected. These patients, often from diverse racial and cultural backgrounds, have well-established, and often poor, personal food habits. A positive approach is required to correct misinformation, faulty eating habits, and food idiosyncrasies.

Inadequate Dentition. Few individuals reach old age with a full complement of teeth. Inadequate dentition and ill-fitting, uncomfortable dentures are important contributors to undernutrition. In the absence of good mastication, food normally prepared may be unsuitable. Poor dentition also results in avoidance of foods that require thorough mastication, tending to limit the diet to softer foods. Gradually, important foods are automatically excluded from the diet—especially meats and fresh fruits and vegetables, the normal sources of vitamins and bulk. This results in poor food habits and an unbalanced and poor diet. Oral and dental hygiene and adequate dentition are important in the elderly patient. A dentist should make periodic scheduled visits to the nursing home, each patient being checked at least twice a year.

Social and Economic Factors.   Economic factors significantly modify the food pattern of most elderly people. They tend to eat the cheaper carbohydrate foods and to ignore the nutritionally more important, but also more expensive, protein foods. Packaged bakery goods, which are cheap and require no further preparation, enjoy a popularity among the elderly that does not comport with nutritional well-being. Many elderly people live alone and lack the facilities to prepare meals and keep foods properly. Moreover, such lonely circumstances supply little incentive to organize meals. Some elderly persons have family conflicts and imaginary grievances that are reflected in their refusal to eat properly, while others are physically unable to take care of themselves. Once again, food habits acquired by the elderly person who has been living alone, often with a restricted income and with poor kitchen facilities, follow him into the nursing home.

Habits. Eating habits are one of the greatest obstacles to the establishment of optimal diets among the majority of persons. Habits—good, bad, or indifferent—once acquired, become fixed by repetition. The longer food habits have been established, the more rigid and ingrained they become.

The dietary pattern of many elderly persons is therefore a formidable structure that is difficult to modify; in too many cases it is based on gustatory preference, self-indulgence, prejudice, indifference, lack of appetite, poor fluid intake, apathy, and fear—fear of the "wrong" foods, fear of constipation, or fear of "indigestion." It is also to be remembered that milk, fruits, and vegetables, so widely distributed today, were not readily available when most 70-year-old persons were young and were forming their personal food habits.

Psychological Factors. In the elderly the value of food and eating is often increased; it is their one remaining source of real pleasure. Although a *decreased* food intake may be one of the first symptoms of physical illness, it may also be due to emotional depression. A mild decrease of food intake in the passive individual may be due to his underactive, underinterested make-up and needs no particular attention; by contrast, in the emotionally depressed a similar decrease might signal the beginning of a serious emotional disturbance, indicating that he is subject to such delusions as a belief that he is unworthy, with no right to food, or that the food is poisoned. Some persons avoid certain foods about which they hold superstitions or obsessions. As long as the avoidance of a particular food does not impair nutritional intake, there is no reason for concern, and it is not necessary to urge its acceptance.

Increased food intake may also be the forerunner of emotional upset. Overeating that is merely a continuance of a life-long pattern will not be of significance. However, overeating because of obsession, delusions, or as a means of relieving anxiety may be helped by substituting other interests. Although overeating can bring on the gastrointestinal symptoms of heartburn, cramps, nausea, and diarrhea, a patient's complaints about the digestibility of food are often evidence of emotional disturbance. Complaints of this nature are frequently used to gain special consideration, to control the food situation, or merely to avoid disliked foods. Dietary habits are influenced markedly by their psychological significance, largely unrelated to the act of eating and the relationships involved in the consumption of food. Symbolic meanings of food dating from his early development affect the food pattern of the individual. Alterations in food intake are sometimes indicative of anxieties.

Mealtime can be especially lonely for the elderly, who often feel rejected by their family and friends. When these patients were young, meals were a time not only for eating, but also for family conviviality. Therefore, whenever possible, ambulatory and wheelchair patients should have their meals together in the dining room. The attractiveness of the meal, cheerful service, and pleasant surroundings all serve as psychological boosts for these elderly people. The well-decorated dining room, with flowers and bright colorful tablecloths, can greatly enhance the attractiveness of a meal.

Well-prepared meals of good nutritional content can still seem drab in the absence of cheerful surroundings and pleasant service.

Physiological Factors. With advancing age there is a diminishing sensitivity to taste and smell that interferes with the normal pleasure associated with eating. The secretion of hydrochloric acid in the stomach and of digestive enzymes in general also diminishes; indeed, the total volume of secretions of the gastrointestinal tract decreases. Digestion and absorption therefore may not be optimal in many elderly persons.

Biliary impairment, which is often present, interferes with normal digestion and utilization of fats and may result in flatulence and discomfort after the ingestion of fatty foods. Stores of the fat-soluble vitamins may decrease, either because of voluntary abstention from fats and the associated fat-soluble vitamins or because of poor intestinal absorption resulting from biliary insufficiency. Constipation, about which the elderly frequently complain, is rarely a result of diet or, as often believed, a physiological debility consequent on aging. Bowel function, however, is greatly affected by decreased muscle tone, low fluid intake, reliance on laxatives, diminished physical activity, and the avoidance of fruits and vegetables, the normal source of bulk. Complaints of constipation that are confirmed by observed bowel habits should, of course, be reported to the physician, since constipation in this age group is frequently an early symptom of bowel cancer.

There tends to be a negative nitrogen balance in old age as the dietary protein intake diminishes and nitrogen assimilation becomes less efficient, while the catabolism of tissue protein slowly increases. The ill effects of hypoproteinemia—wound repair, predisposition to anemia, and decreased resistance to infection—are thus more conspicuous in advanced age.

CALORIC IMBALANCE. Since the basal metabolic rate decreases in old age, fewer calories are needed to satisfy the body energy required for the upkeep of its vital functions. Paralleling the drop in metabolic rate, physical activity also decreases, thus diminishing considerably the total caloric requirement. Nevertheless, in too many aging persons their previous eating habits persist, despite the marked reduction in energy expenditure. Obesity increases surgical risk, predisposes to cardiovascular disease, and has a deleterious effect on the weight-bearing joints in osteoarthritis. Actually, because of the increased incidence of degenerative disease among the obese and their shorter life span, overweight is not a common problem among the truly aged. Among septuagenarians and octogenarians, caloric deprivation and emaciation are more prevalent than obesity. On the other hand, extreme underweight and undernutrition are equally undesirable. Adjustment of the caloric intake and body weight of the elderly person must therefore be one of the basic objectives of a sound geriatric nutritional regimen.

VITAMIN AND MINERAL REQUIREMENTS. Inasmuch as the vitamin requirement is not markedly changed in old age, greater attention must be paid to an adequate dietary supply, since a diminished total food intake, poor qualitative selection of food items, and possibly less efficient absorption set the stage for vitamin deficiencies. The lack of vitamins affects many tissues and organs in the body and may lead to serious disease. Calcium and iron intakes are likely to be insufficient. The occurrence of chronic iron-deficiency anemia is associated with the diminished secretion of gastric hydrochloric acid.

In the past, the frequency of osteoporosis (demineralization of bones) and fractures among the elderly was attributed to low calcium intakes. Actually osteoporosis is the result of many factors. With a decreased secretion of the body hormones, there is less elaboration of the bone matrix. An adequate protein intake and a positive calcium balance are essential for the prevention of osteoporosis. Parathyroid-hormone deficiencies also contribute to the demineralization of bone. It is clear that the provision of an adequate nutritional diet cannot be haphazard; it requires the help and advice of physicians and dieticians. Small nursing homes should cooperate to share the services of a dietician or some other person who is trained in nutrition to supervise their programs.

DIETARY RECOMMENDATIONS

In view of the preceding considerations, some dietary recommendations can be made. The optimum diet in later years should be high in proteins, moderate in carbohydrates, relatively low in fats, and rich in vitamins and minerals. The total caloric intake should suffice to maintain a body weight consistent with, or slightly below, that which was normal for the individual at the age of 25. Any existing overweight or underweight should be corrected gradually.

The intake of fats should be less than 30 per cent of the total caloric intake. In advanced age about 25 per cent of the caloric intake should come from fat. The diet should be rich in all vitamins and minerals since in old age less of these substances are absorbed; supplements can be provided. Sufficient iron and calcium should be offered to correct existing deficiencies and to maintain normal balance.

The fluid intake should be 6 to 8 glasses daily. Sufficient liquids should be consumed to permit excretion of at least 1.5 liters of urine per day; this requires a daily intake of about 2 quarts of fluid. A liberal intake of water, juices, milk, coffee, and tea, spaced throughout the day, helps to maintain a normal flow of urine and counteracts tendencies to constipation. The stimulating effect of caffeine in coffee and tea is not harmful, except in specific illnesses. When insomnia is a problem, coffee or tea late in the day should be avoided. The moderate use of alcoholic beverages is often regarded as helpful in the nutritional care of the aged—for example, a glass of wine before dinner often increases a lagging appetite and has a vasodilating effect; its relaxing properties are also valuable at bedtime.

A large proportion of patients who have been placed on salt-restricted diets because of cardiovascular disorders are in the older age group. In these persons salt depletion during hot weather is possible, but rarely encountered.

The elderly do not willingly accept abrupt changes. To avoid emotional disturbance and outright rejection of advice, any changes in diet should be gradual and should be suited to the individual as far as possible. For example, fluid milk is rejected by many aged persons; dried skim milk introduced into customary foods will often prove acceptable and avoid such mealtime problems.

When chewing is difficult, ground or chopped meat or tender fish is preferable; soft fruits or juices are best substituted for hard fruits. The emphasis should turn to egg or cheese dishes, finely chopped vegetables, and puddings and soups which may be enriched with milk or dry-milk solids. Strained and junior infant foods, which require no preparation, present a large selection of nutritious items.

Therapeutic Diets. In a nursing home special therapeutic diets involve many individuals: the administrator, the physician, the person planning the therapeutic diet, the person planning the regular menu, the person purchasing food and supplies, the cook who prepares the diet, the nurse's aide who serves the diet, the aide who observes the food eaten by the patient, and the patient's family. If no dietician is available, the professional nurse is best prepared to coordinate, orient, and provide inservice training in preparing and serving a therapeutic diet to nursing-home patients. Professional nurses must be well informed about the therapeutic diets most commonly prescribed, since they alone are competent to exercise the careful attention and supervision needed. The administrator should be informed of special needs in order to establish policies and to buy supplies and equipment.

A nursing home is justified in limiting the variety of different diets it can serve. When the physician prescribes a type of diet, the nurse on duty should show the physician which diet used by the home will be selected as a guide in planning his patient's meals. If the physician is not satisfied with the diet offered, he should provide an outline of the diet to be used. To ease the workload on the kitchen staff, the modified menus should be as similar to the regular menu as possible. When the person planning the menu is informed about the variety of diets needed and the restrictions these diets impose, the regular menu can be planned to provide foods suitable for many of the modified diets. This is not to say that all foods should be prepared without salt, fat, sugar, or spices because of the restriction of a few. It does mean that main dishes, vegetables, salads, and desserts can be varied from day to day and coordinated so that the food is properly prepared and seasoned to meet the tastes and needs of each individual in the nursing home without unduly burdening the kitchen staff with the preparation of dozens of extra items.

Advance planning is the key to efficient food-service management and is particularly important for serving therapeutic diets. A written menu for each kind of diet ensures accuracy in preparation and serving. The therapeutic diets, like all institutional diets, should be imaginatively written to avoid monotony. When modified diets are planned in advance, any extra foods needed can be purchased with the regular food orders, and the cook can have all food items correctly prepared at the time the meal is served. Such planning can eliminate the use of the substitute special pack foods which may not be as appetizing.

To guarantee that the patient always receives the correct diet, all diets served should be identified with the patient's name and location. Tray cards of different colors help the staff to recognize a modified diet. The staff requires orientation and inservice training to avoid mistakes such as giving salt to a patient on a sodium-restricted diet or sugar to a diabetic patient.

Diets are for people, not for diseases. As far as possible, the patient should be informed about his diet so that he can understand and accept it. He may not be happy with it, but he is more likely to accept it if he understands it. The ultimate success of diet therapy rests upon the cooperation of the patient and the support and encouragement he receives from the staff and his family.

Administrative Aspects

FOOD SANITATION

Clean surroundings and sanitary procedures in the handling and preparation of foods are essential. The nursing home is obligated to offer food that is nutritious, prepared and served attractively, and sanitary.

Food Poisoning. The end result of unsanitary or unsafe food-handling techniques can be food poisoning. The types of food poisoning with which one is most likely to be concerned are:

1. Chemical food poisoning. Cleaning supplies, insecticides, and all nonfood items must be labeled and kept away from foods.
2. Botulism. This occurs infrequently and usually in prepared and canned foods, where it cannot be identified. However, if the can has been damaged the food should not be used. A can that bulges outward usually means spoiled food.
3. *Staphylococcus* infection. This is caused by contamination by staphylococci. The usual symptoms are vomiting, which is usually projectile, and diarrhea. The onset is from 2 to 4 hours after ingestion of the food.

4. *Salmonella* infection. This is a food infection caused by ingestion of the *Salmonella* bacillus. The symptoms are severe abdominal cramps, diarrhea, vomiting, fever, and chills. It is important to note that these pathogenic bacteria give no warning because they cause no change in the taste, appearance, or odor of food. Growth of bacteria can be controlled by proper personal hygiene, sanitary food-handling procedures, exposure to heat above 140°F. or destruction by chemicals—for example, chlorine, iodine, or other proved sanitizers applied to utensils after ordinary cleaning.

Personal Hygiene. Personnel who handle food should be clean and in a good state of health. They should wear clean, washable garments and a suitable hair covering. No food handler should be permitted to work with infected cuts or burns or when suffering from an upper-respiratory-tract infection—spray from a sneeze may be projected as far as 15 feet or more. Frequent inspection of food handlers at work is necessary, and regular classes of instruction should be instituted to teach basic sanitary principles. Since they are the most frequent sources of transmission of bacteria to foods, hands should be washed thoroughly and frequently. Food should be handled as little as possible.

Care of Food. All prepared food, whether hot or cold, should be kept covered and at the correct temperature during preparation and all waiting periods. All ready-to-eat foods should be covered during storage and transportation. In addition to guarding against contamination, covering food keeps it in a better state

—moister, fresher in color, crisper, and generally more attractive and appealing when served.

TIME AND TEMPERATURE. The ideal temperature for incubation of bacteria is 45 to 150° F. Therefore, ready-to-eat foods should be kept below or above this range. The length of time that food is held over is important. Production should be geared to actual anticipated amount to be used to cut leftovers to a minimum. If at all possible, food should be consumed within 24 hours after preparation. The use of a water bath for holding food after it has been prepared should be prohibited. Many cook's tables are equipped with a *bain-marie* to enable the cook to prepare food in advance and keep it warm until ready to serve. Tests have shown that too often the temperature falls below 150° F., making it an unsafe method for holding foods, especially milk products, meats, and sauces. Food poisoning develops easily in protein foods, especially those kept in this manner for an hour or more. Cooks must be trained to time the cooking so that food will be finished as close to the actual serving time as possible. Steam tables are not recommended for holding food, since they often present the same problem as the *bain-marie*. In order to prevent burns from the steam, cooks often turn the heat down; the temperature of the food, which is often uncovered, then falls below the safe 150° F. Electric dry-heat counters and food carts are recommended; they are safer and much more satisfactory.

SELECTION OF EQUIPMENT

The following questions are suggested when new items of equipment are being considered: What is the need? What should the piece of equipment do? What limitations are there on a selection—(e.g., budget, space, power, operation, and maintenance)? Will the use justify the expenditure, the space occupied, and the time required for cleaning and care? Is the item simple to operate? Is it sanitary and easy to clean and maintain? Is it standard? Have all types and sources of such items been investigated to ensure the best selection?

The *need* should be clearly defined. The various kinds of equipment available to do the same kind of a job should be studied; often one type can do several jobs. Balance the need for an item against other needs. Do not be influenced by the ideas of a single person, who may not have a complete understanding of the overall operation and appropriateness of the equipment. The limitations of a piece of new equipment must be defined as plans are developed and decisions made. A study should be made to be certain that adequate space is available, that the item will not make other work inconvenient, that it is conveniently located, and that it can be easily cleaned. It is important to know that a prospective piece of equipment is simple to use and is sanitary. A national organization, the National Sanitation Foundation, undertakes to evaluate food-service utensils. The organization's main evaluation are the sanitary features. Any equipment or utensils that have been inspected and approved carry a NSF seal that can be used as a guide for purchasing equipment. Incidentally, if cost is not a serious factor, stainless steel equipment should always be considered.

FOOD PURCHASING

In general, one should plan at least a week or two in advance in order to purchase effectively. Purchasing should always be done on a competitive basis. Any one can develop a standard sheet that will show what is to be purchased, with a column for quotations from two or three dealers. It is helpful to develop a guide in setting up specifications to indicate grade and quality desired. The American Hospital Association publishes *A Food Purchasing Guide, Manual for Specification of Canned Fruits and Vegetables.* The Hospital section of the Connecticut State Department of Health has a Diet Manual and a Food Service Manual for diet planning and food purchasing.

10
Physical Therapy in Rehabilitation

————— ◆•◆ —————

Pʜʏsɪᴄᴀʟ therapy is defined in Blakiston's New
Gould Medical (Second Edition) as "the treatment of
disease and injury by physical means . . . performed by
trained personnel under the prescription of a physician."
Rehabilitation is the restoration of an ill or injured
patient to self-sufficiency or to gainful employment at
his highest attainable skill in the shortest possible time.
Rehabilitation therapy may be defined as assisting the
patient by all available physical and emotional means
to be as independent as possible within the realistic
limits of his disability. The emotional factor is emphasized because, in dealing with geriatric patients in
nursing homes, one encounters both psychological and
physical impairment. We shall therefore consider more
than the mere modalities of physical therapy. The prin-
cipal aim of physical rehabilitation of the geriatric patient is to endow him, not only with the highest possible degree of physical independence within the nurs-

ing home but also, whenever possible, with sufficient independence to allow him to return to his family, to a "foster home," or to independent living. Successful achievement of this goal, even if only partial, not only benefits the patient but also lightens the work load for the nursing-home personnel.

Activities of daily living (ADL), for example, are important in any discussion of rehabilitation. The following is an enlightening quotation from *Physical Rehabilitation for Daily Living*: "ADL means activities of daily living, or as a patient once said, 'All the little things that make you miserable when you cannot do them—you know, like putting on your shoes, or eating your soup, or switching on the light, or getting from the bed to the wheelchair or walking through a door.' They are little things, to be sure, but if one is on braces and crutches they become strenuous exercises. They assume utmost importance, because when they are all added up, they make the difference between constantly needing help and being on one's own."

This quotation provides an important guide to geriatric rehabilitation. Little things *are* important. It must be recognized that gains in function that seem small and insignificant to a normal healthy person may represent a great achievement to the disabled patient. For example, by teaching a patient to feed himself, one raises him from the status of a dependent infant, enables him to eat at his own pace, and select the foods he prefers. Eating can again become enjoyable to a patient who has achieved this degree of independence. Furthermore, one cannot forget the economic importance of such functional achievement; the patient who is able to feed himself no longer needs the personal attendance of a member of the staff at each meal. Thus, successful rehabilitation leads both to independence for the patient and to a reduction in the cost of care. Little things are, indeed, important!

Personnel Involved in Rehabilitation

Ideally a rehabilitation program is directed by a physiatrist who has physical therapists, occupational therapists, educational therapists, and speech therapists available to implement the program. Psychologists, social service personnel, consulting physicians, and nursing personnel are also necessary for the ideal rehabilitation program. However, such staffing is usually available only in specialized rehabilitation institutes. Chronic hospitals, convalescent hospitals, and nursing homes do not have the economic resources to provide such staffing patterns. Even the best chronic hospitals that have departments in all of the above-named specialties often maintain only token staffs in many of the departments. Furthermore, there are insufficient numbers of trained therapists even when funds to pay their salaries and maintenance are available.

However, lack of specially trained personnel does not mean that programs of geriatric rehabilitation cannot be initiated in the nursing home. Significant degrees of success can be achieved by adhering to the principles outlined below. Consulting services from the rehabilitation departments of a local, and preferably affiliated, hospital will still be required in guiding the programs and in providing advice on special problems, but practical programs can be started with a modest staff.

In dealing with the chronically disabled geriatric patient there are several points that must be kept in mind. One must avoid the pitfall of being frustrated too easily. For various reasons, these patients have considerable difficulty attaining certain functions. If one's frustration is transmitted to the patient, one may actually prevent him from making the gains that are within his physical capabilities.

One cannot love each and every patient. Many people have personalities that are antagonistic, and they exhibit these traits in sickness as well as health. If one allows oneself to feel a sense of guilt over harboring dislike toward a certain type of patient, one can fall into one of two pitfalls: one avoids the patient and neglects to provide the care he requires, or one becomes oversolicitous in an attempt to win him over. In either case, the patient's progress in rehabilitation will probably be impeded. If one can face the fact that patients differ temperamentally, one can learn to treat them equally despite their idiosyncracies, facilitating the task of rehabilitation for both patient and therapist.

One must also recognize the reverse; it can be disastrous to make a "pet" of a patient. It is all too easy to give too much attention to personable patients or to those who have pleasant families. In such cases, for example, one may find oneself offering assistance to the patient who is slow in self-feeding and allows his food to get cold or giving a patient a bed bath because of the difficulty he experiences in bathing himself in a tub. As a result, the patient soon becomes dependent upon such assistance instead of developing the independence of which he is capable.

The families of patients must be brought into these

programs; they must be made aware of rehabilitation goals. It is extremely important that they understand the objectives of a program so that they do not misinterpret the actions taken. Most families are receptive to joining in a program for functional improvement of the patient, but if they do not understand the objectives, they may come into the institution and deal with the patient in ways that set back all efforts at rehabilitation.

Setting Realistic Goals

Realistic goals must be set when one is establishing rehabilitation objectives. This rule applies to any type of institution. The goals must be realistic from the standpoint not only of the patient's capabilities but also of available personnel and treatment facilities. In the aged patient it is more desirable to set a limited goal that can be raised at a later date than to establish an aim that is unattainable and can only frustrate the patient and those who are trying to rehabilitate him.

FOR AMPUTEES

Several examples can be cited to illustrate this point. The geriatric patient who has had an above-knee amputation should not be led to think that he will be as nimble and secure on a prosthesis as he was on his own leg. It is better to have the patient recognize that it will be most difficult to manage ambulation on a prosthesis. It is usually helpful to warn the patient of the difficulties that he will encounter, so that each achievement will be a victory. The patient will be trying to walk on a device that does not provide the sensations of motion, touch and proprioception afforded by the normal leg. Consequently, he does not know where the limb is when he first starts to use it and thus lacks the security of orientation.

FOR HEMIPLEGICS

In hemiplegic patients this problem of establishing realistic goals is very important. Although the patient should not be discouraged to the point of initiating immobility and the development of contractures, it may be unwise to allow him to think that he will walk immediately and be completely independent. While this may be the hoped-for objective, it may be unattainable for even the best-motivated patient. He should take each step in functional rehabilitation in its proper order. He should first be encouraged to feed and dress himself and perform other functions that do not require walking. Even these will require considerable work and assistance.

The example of hemiplegic patients is mentioned because many patients with this disability do not walk well even though they have sufficient apparent muscle strength to perform this action. Usually such a patient is labeled as being poorly motivated or is even thought to be a malingerer. In many cases, however, these patients have neurological deficits that are less obvious than the easily recognized disabilitites of paralysis or aphasia.

FOR AGNOSIA PATIENTS

Agnosia, the loss of ability to recognize the import of sensory stimuli, is one such deficit. In a recent case, a 52-year-old man sustained a left-sided hemiplegia after a cerebral thrombosis three and a half years before. Following that episode, the patient was provided with a brace, and after several months of therapy was able to ambulate. He was discharged home, where he was content to sit in a wheelchair. He was readmitted two years later with contractures of the knee and hip, which were relieved by intensive therapy. It was then found that the patient was unable to recognize stimuli on the involved side when both legs were tested simultaneously; the patient could not feel his left leg and appreciate where it was when he walked. Consequently, he refused to walk because he was frightened by not knowing where his leg was in relation to his body. When he was provided with a walker, the support provided by that device enabled him to improve measurably.

FOR APRAXIA PATIENTS

Apraxia, the loss of the previously acquired ability to perform intricate skilled acts, is another source of great difficulty. In this case the patient knows what he wants to do, but may not be able to accomplish the act. With apraxia of speech, he may speak in a gibberish because he cannot say the proper words; with motor apraxia, a part of the body refuses to function normally. A patient with a motor apraxia may have difficulty walking because his leg refuses to obey his commands, although he may have good strength in the individual muscles of the affected limb. Unless one is aware of the true nature of the disability, it is easy to reject such a patient as a malingerer.

Autotopagnosia is a more extreme degree of agnosia

in which the patient loses the ability to localize or orient correctly different parts of the body. A patient with this defect may even have difficulty in sitting straight in a wheelchair; he has an annoying tendency to fall to one side. Straps or specially placed pillows may be required to keep the patient upright; in other cases, foot pedals with web heel loops will enable him to sit properly in the chair. Once the patient is helped to remain upright, he may achieve a considerable degree of independence in a chair.

It is recognized that untrained personnel will be unable to make the diagnosis of such disabilities; however, since they deal with large numbers of geriatric patients who are prone to such problems, they must be made aware of their experience. Such awareness will help in setting proper goals for patients and, more important, in realizing that goals must be changed as one's knowledge of patients grows.

It must be emphasized that one should, of course, work for the highest level of function possible in each patient, but one must recognize that various factors play a role in determining what that level may be. If it is realized that little things are important, one will take each step in its proper order and not attempt to accomplish the entire program in one leap. Such attempts too often lead to failure.

Knowing the Patient

In order to plan a proper therapeutic program for any patient, it is important to know him as a person.

This seems so elementary as hardly to justify mention. However, lack of familiarity with patients as persons is a major shortcoming in modern medicine. Although physicians may know more about the chemistry and bodily affinity for isotopes of their patients than before, there appears on their charts little information to identify these patients, their occupations, and their abilities.

One must know a patient's racial background, religion, hobbies, family ties, occupation, and home situation. Information about a patient's race, for example, will allow a dietician to prescribe a special diet to which the patient may adhere. A patient of Italian descent, for example, may go off his diet because he dislikes macaroni and cheese cooked according to an American recipe. Slight adjustments in menu based on such information will gain his cooperation, with successful therapeutic results.

Knowledge of hobbies and occupation directs one in helping the patient regain the function necessary for a vocational rehabilitation. The occupational therapist has a much easier time if the activities prescribed are adapted to the patient's previous habits. If his religion is known, this knowledge can often be used to motivate the patient.

Proper planning for a patient's future depends very much upon the physical structure of his home. For example, one must know if a patient must go up and down stairs. Measurement of doorway width may determine the type of wheelchair that must be ordered for a patient. Who else lives at home and what is their physical status? These are some of the facts that one must know to evaluate when the patient may be discharged to home.

Rehabilitation Treatment

PHYSICAL THERAPY

Physical therapy of significant degree can be administered by qualified nurses in almost all cases. Expert supervision may be necessary in complicated cases, and in most cases the physician in charge should supervise the overall exercise program. In most cases, however, this need not be considered a prerequisite; common sense is the necessary ingredient of a successful program, provided certain basic principles are remembered.

In general, active exercise is more desirable than passive exercise. This is easily understood if it is recognized that the average patient will limit the range of motion at the point where pain occurs. The onset of pain warns him when damage might follow. This is a point that is of special significance following surgical procedures for orthopedic problems. Active exercise has the benefits of improving circulation and reducing stasis edema. When active exercise includes weight bearing, the additional benefit of positive calcium balance may be achieved.

When passive exercise is necessary, common sense can direct what that exercise should be. In exercising a paralyzed limb of a patient, for example, one can determine the type of exercise and the limits of joint motion by simply observing the normal ranges in a normal limb. To do this, one needs only observe one's own arm or leg. If resistance is encountered in passive exercise, it is a simple warning to proceed with care. If signs such as crepitus are elicited, the exercise should not be repeated except on expert advice. It is worthy of note that passive exercise involves more than the therapist's activity. If a knee and thigh can be kept supple, a patient can continue to get up in a wheelchair. The patient who does not have contractures can be kept more comfortable and does not require special beds. Pressure lesions can also be more easily avoided when there are no contractures.

Heat may be applied for therapeutic effects in any situation in which it may be indicated. Warm, moist packs or a gooseneck lamp with a standard bulb may provide the heat source, provided it is not so hot as to cause burns. Heat is useful in relieving pain and may help in reducing spasm. Expensive devices are not always necessary.

Hydrotherapy is available wherever there are washbasins and bathtubs. Painful arthritic hands can often be relieved simply by bathing them in a basin of warm water. Bathing in a warm tub provides more extensive hydrotherapy, and is not an unreasonable substitute for a Hubbard tank. Interestingly enough, most persons who take it for granted that soaking in a hot tub is soothing to a few aches and pains after a day of strenuous work are often reluctant to provide the same therapy for a patient unless they have a special prescription.

SPECIAL DEVICES

Special but simple devices can be improvised for disabled patients, many of whom require only simple aids rather than complex mechanisms. One can improvise eating utensils with large handles for the patient with a poor grip simply by taping wooden blocks to standard utensils. A combination knife and fork is obviously helpful for the patient with use of only one hand. The wheelchair-bound patient with use of only one arm should have a one-arm-drive chair. Such a chair can be driven by two rims on the "good arm" side; these can operate both wheels simultaneously and allow the patient to travel in a straight line rather than in circles. The wheelchair patient who uses his feet to propel his chair may benefit by having the pedals removed so that he does not continually bump his ankles. The bilateral amputee patient should have an amputee chair with offset axles that change the center of gravity so that he does not tip over. The patient who has difficulty in shifting out of a wheelchair should have a chair with removable sidearms.

Other simple devices can be provided without special consultation. The patient who is developing flexion deformity at the wrist should be supplied with a simple cock-up splint. If a patient is developing flexion deformity at the knee, a simple extension splint may be made with rolls of newspaper and a blanket. The patient with a paralyzed arm and a painful shoulder will usually feel considerable relief if he is provided with an arm sling. Paraplegic patients can help themselves if they have a bed trapeze and straps attached to the foot of the bed which they can use to pull themselves to a sitting position.

CLOTHING

Even a superficial discussion of rehabilitation requires mention of the value of having patients wear their own clothes whenever possible. It is depressing to patients to keep them in institutional pajamas and robes if they are really candidates for rehabilitation. It is to be remembered that the patient can be rehabilitated for both institutional living and discharge. It is not normal for anyone to spend his life in pajamas; wearing one's own clothes provides an important element of identity and independence. It has also been observed that many patients show remarkable improvement in incontinence when they wear their own clothes; obviously, a person is less inclined to soil his own clothing if he has any degree of sphincter control.

An Illustrative Case

A 38-year-old married shipyard worker, the father of four children, was admitted to the hospital two months following hospitalization for one month at another institution for a craniotomy involving a ruptured aneurysm. The patient was on an acute service for seven weeks before being transferred to the intermediate service. At the time of transfer, the doctor's and nurse's notes indicated that the patient was mute, quadriparetic, and unresponsive and would not feed himself. He had a sacral decubitus. The chart indicated that the patient had little prognosis for anything more than a vegetative existence.

The patient was transferred to the intermediate service in the morning. The attending physician did not examine him until early afternoon, at which time he was told by the nurse that the patient could talk and could feed himself. The patient was sitting up in a wheelchair with a padded cushion. He could indeed talk, knew that he had four children and gave their names, although he did not remember their correct ages. He also explained accurately what his job had been.

The nurses asked if they could try to "push" the patient to see what he could do, and they were given permission to do so. The nursing staff then accomplished the following: on the evening of transfer the patient walked with minimal assistance; he continued to feed himself; he was able to wheel a chair about the ward; and he was continent of urine during the day. On the second day, he played cards with other patients, who were encouraged to help him; during the second game he arranged his cards properly and played his suits in order.

These things were accomplished in forty-eight hours. Dedicated nurses had apparently performed a miracle in a man who had a prognosis of little hope. Actually, the nurses had not performed a miracle; they had only shown interest in the patient and given him the chance to show what he could do. He had previously been mute because no one had bothered to talk to him. This case may represent the dramatic extreme, but it illustrates what can be done by nursing personnel who are interested and given some latitude.

Conclusion

Rehabilitation is often considered to be a very complicated affair requiring the utmost in modern physical facilities. Unfortunately, most nursing homes have very little in the way of special facilities, while they have an abundance of disabled patients in need of rehabilitative therapy. Rehabilitation, however, can be accomplished by anyone who has the desire. Most nurses can apply common sense and do a reasonably competent job in rehabilitation if only they have the time.

The field of rehabilitation is not as dramatic as many other areas of medicine. Television and the news media have accustomed us to the wonderful world of mechanics in medicine: if a patient does not require an open-heart operation, an artificial kidney, or an organ transplant, he is not considered to be very interesting. The truth is that rehabilitation and good nursing care primarily require personal attention to the patient and to basic principles of good medicine. Accolades are not given for the results achieved in this type of work; no one will read in the headlines about a stroke patient learning to walk. The rewards are to be found only in the satisfaction of accomplishment and in the gratitude of the patient.

11
Hearing

———— •••• ————

THE ability to communicate is one of the most important functions in life, for a person without this capacity withdraws into himself. His living experiences become limited, his personality may change so that he appears dull when he is not, and his world of sound is relived only through memories. In elderly patients, who comprise most of the nursing-home population and who are limited in so many ways, the maintenance of two-way communication is particularly important. Life is difficult for the elderly; it is hard for them to learn how to cope with problems and to adjust to experiences even less drastic than that of deafness. It is therefore all the more vital that these people be aided to maintain some degree of hearing as long as possible. Thus, a hearing program becomes an essential part of rehabilitation therapy.

Therapy for Deafness

The deterioration of the hearing mechanism in old people is called presbycusis. The eighth cranial nerve gradually deteriorates, causing increasing loss of hearing. The perception of high-frequency sounds gradually recedes—the higher the frequency, the poorer the hearing. Although otosclerosis occasionally develops, even patients with this disability can hear with the help of a hearing aid because they have been able to adjust gradually to their impairment and have learned to live with diminished hearing.

Persons who begin to have hearing loss after the age of 65 have the symptoms of presbycusis; they should receive help and instruction in lipreading. Thereby they learn exactly how the speech sounds are made and how to form them, and they also learn to make the most of their residual hearing. However, if vision also is impaired, the patient may be unable to lipread; then one must turn to the hearing aid as a substitute.

Many individuals will require both a hearing aid and a knowledge of lipreading. One must assess the individual's abilities carefully. If he has only a mild hearing loss, lipreading should be tried to obviate a dependence on hearing aids. One should not prescribe a hearing aid unless the hearing loss is at least 30 decibels. If the patient has less than this degree of hearing loss, he should first be placed in lipreading classes. If necessary, a hearing aid can always be prescribed, but only as a supplement.

HEARING AIDS

A hearing aid for an elderly patient should be a separate instrument and not one that is attached to his eyeglass frame; if he removes his glasses, he also removes his hearing. Also, it is best to have a minimum number of controls on the aid, since the older patient may throw them out of adjustment. Obviously, hearing aids should not be prescribed for patients in a confused mental condition.

Adjusting to a Hearing Aid. When a patient is considering a hearing aid, he should try one for at least a week. It is difficult to assess the ability of the older person to adapt to and to use such a device. One must take a positive approach toward patients wearing a hearing aid. The patient should never be asked whether he wishes to wear his hearing aid; inevitably, he will refuse to do so. Rather, it should be assumed that he will put it on, as he would a piece of clothing, in preparation for the day's activities. At the outset, a person learning to wear a hearing aid will require help; a person who becomes deaf loses his ability to "not hear" what he does not wish to hear. Thus, after a period of deafness, every sound suddenly is very loud. He hears the tap of every high heel, every click of silverware, and the thud of every door that is closed. The patient should wear the hearing aid for two hours the first day and for three to four hours a day thereafter for a week. Sudden noise is distracting; therefore, before a patient enters a noisy dining room he should have worn the hearing aid for three or four days in quieter situations.

Some people adjust very readily to a hearing aid and never need to remove it once they have accustomed themselves to it. If a patient cannot wear it all day at the end of two or three weeks, he will have difficulty, for this indicates that he has not regained the ability to hear only what he wishes to hear. However, a patient's failure to adjust readily need not be a cause for despair. With patience and practice one may be able to help even the slow patient. While patients should never be compelled to wear a hearing aid, one can and should try very hard to convince them that they should use such a device even if they are having difficulty in adjusting to it or are beginning to have emotional problems.

Reading as an Adjunct.   Once patients begin to wear hearing aids, the instructor should read to them, and they should read to each other. Newspapers are especially good, since the captions are large. The patient is at an advantage when he is with someone who has the same problem. When patients both realize how loud a slammed door sounds, they appreciate their mutual problems. It is important to teach a beginner to watch the person who is speaking, although persons with normal vision usually do this naturally. Obviously, a person wearing a hearing aid or with a hearing handicap will hear more if he watches the speaker.

LIPREADING

Lipreading is extremely important as an adjunct to speech to a hard-of-hearing person. He must learn to say those things that are most useful to him. If he is able to speak, he is able to make his wants known. With beginning lipreaders, start by teaching them that the P, B, and M sounds are made in the same fashion—that is, with the lips together. There is no other way to make a pa, ba, and ma sound.

Then, with lips together, familiarize them with the way the sounds are made and which ones may look alike. Start with the words *before, best,* and *butter.* First, display these words to them so that they can see them;

then turn and face them so that they see you say *before,* *best,* and *butter.* The next three words are *blue, bring,* and *better.* In a beginning class, all of the sentences should have the word *before* in them and no other word with a similar sound. For example, "Close the window *before* you go." "*Before* you close the window, put up the shade." "It might rain *before* you return." The next words are *best, blue,* and *butter.* For example, "This is my *best* dress." "My *best* dress is navy *blue* with a white collar and cuffs." "I take good care of it because it is my *best* dress." "Please *butter* my toast for me." "I like toast hot so that the *butter* melts." "The sky is getting *blue* today." "I like *blue* sky with white fluffy clouds." "The clearer the *blue,* the *better* I like it." "*Bring* me the coat in the living room." "If you forget your coat, I will *bring* it down for you." Then use a word starting with the letter P. For example, "*Please* decide you will mend this yourself." When patients miss a word go back over it and help them with it until they understand increasing numbers of words. Later, write a word on the blackboard and enunciate it without sound. Use current topics—holidays, gatherings, and contemporary happenings—for material. Read something very short to the patients and then ask them questions about the material you have read. Try to communicate the main idea; if there are any questions, go over the material again and make conversation. This is an exceptionally good way to teach.

In conclusion, the continuity of a hearing program is important; classes should be held at least three times a week, with a volunteer reading, if steady improvement is to be expected. The instructor can develop lipreading material from the magazines. A magazine with pictures is very helpful; select the pictures and use the main captions. The instructor must stimulate his students, make them watch him, make them think, and avoid boring them. A patient who is completely deaf is rare; this usually occurs only with those who have never heard. Most patients have heard speech and imitated it and learned it. Even if he has severe impairment, but speaks words that can be understood, technically a patient is not deaf.

One of the most important things the physician and the nursing staff can do is to encourage the hard-of-hearing to communicate. The remaining days of the elderly should be as happy as possible. When the hard-of-hearing patient learns once more to communicate, he has taken another step forward in his rehabilitation program.

12
Speech Therapy

———◆◆◆———

M ANY patients in nursing homes possess speech disorders. These will vary from mild cases of poor articulation, characterized by the substitution, omission, addition, and distortion of speech sounds, to stroke patients with severe aphasia, loss of the power of speech. Patients who have undergone a laryngectomy may also be seen.

The patient with a speech disorder presents a definite handicap both to himself and to the nursing staff who care for him. It is important for the patient's nurse to be able, not only to recognize the speech disorder, but also to render appropriate support to the rehabilitation program. When the patient's speech is severely limited or when it is distorted, his verbal disability may hinder other aspects of the rehabilitation program. His inability to tell his physician and his nurse how he feels may pose a major problem. By observing his actions, the patient's nurse may interpret what the patient may be trying to communicate; in some cases, he will attempt to communicate through pantomime. It is important for the nurse to encourage the patient to use verbal language as much as possible and not to depend on pointing or pantomiming. The nursing supervisor should be insistent in her instructions that the patient attempt to communicate verbally to the best of his ability every day.

A speech rehabilitation program should be initiated when it is first discovered that the patient has a speech problem. If the patient regresses in his total ability to communicate verbally before speech rehabilitation is begun, this regression may prevent him from achieving the maximum possible progress. In order to prevent this regression, the interactions of the nurse-patient-doctor-therapist relationship should be considered if an understanding, knowledgeable therapeutic program for the patient is to be achieved.

Anatomy and Physiology

The nurse working with the patient with a speech disorder should understand certain elements of speech production. To gain a better understanding of this it is important to consider the speaking system: the vocal folds, the larynx, and the resonating system. The breathing mechanism plays a key role in voice production. The lungs, windpipe, and the walls of the chest cage that cause the chest to expand and contract compose this system. The breathing mechanism furnishes the air pressure required to make the vocal folds vibrate. The vibratory, opening-closing movement of the vocal folds produces a tone. Adjustments in the larynx and the air pressure in the trachea enable the tone to be raised or lowered in pitch and increased or decreased in loudness. The vocal sound can be resonated in the throat and head cavities—mainly in the pharynx and mouth and, in the case of nasal sounds, in the nose cavities. The vocal quality depends, not only on the way in which the vocal folds vibrate, but also on the characteristics of the resonating cavities—that is, their shape, size, and the way the muscular walls and the openings of the particular cavities are adjusted. Adjustments of the openings and sizes of the throat, mouth, and nose help produce the different speech sounds.

When the brain is damaged, a speech disorder may result. The speech center is situated in the third left frontal convolution; some authorities regard Broca's center on this convolution as the speech center. Much is now known of the relationship between damage to certain association areas and defects in speech and understanding of words, but there is a great deal to be learned before discordant theories are reconciled.

Problems of cerebral localization are complicated when correlations are attempted between specific functions of communication and particular cortical areas of the brain. Although it is generally agreed that the formulation of expressive language pertains mainly to Broca's area and that impressive language perception is based in Wernicke's area, the further kinds of symbolic and syntactical communication are not to be strictly ascribed to certain limited centers. When the speech area in the brain is damaged and aphasia results, the nurse caring for the patient should have a basic understanding of the cause of the speech problem and how it can be helped.

Aphasia

PATHOLOGY

Because of its energy requirements, the brain receives over one fifth of the blood pumped from the heart. If the circulation to an area in the brain stops because of hemorrhage or thrombosis, a stroke results. The speech impediment usually associated with the stroke patient is aphasia. Wepman has defined aphasia as any language problem resulting from organic disturbance of cortical brain tissue in which the defect is not caused by faulty nerve impulses to the musculature of speech, loss of function of the peripheral sense organs, or general mental deficiency. The language problem is evidenced by the inability of the individual to use oral or written symbols to express his thoughts and ideas and to transmit them to others.

Types of Aphasia. The commonest types of aphasia are expressive, receptive, and expressive-receptive.

EXPRESSIVE. The patient with expressive aphasia has difficulty in making his thoughts or wants known to others. Writing and speaking are the two aspects of language usually affected. The patient may also have difficulty in reading and understanding speech, but his problem may become evident when he fails to use correct grammar, has difficulty talking on the telephone, and has problems with using appropriate gestures. A patient who was afflicted with a severe expressive aphasia, but had very little receptive difficulty, illustrates this disability. She overheard two nurses discussing her. One of them said, "It's a shame that this girl cannot think and talk; she will never really understand anything." When the nurses were called to a conference, they were given a thorough review of the patient's case history. It was explained that she had expressive and not receptive aphasia. Since she was able to understand everything spoken, such comments by the nurses in the patient's presence were detrimental to her rehabilitation. The nature of expressive aphasia—that is, the patient's inability to express himself, although he understands—should also be explained to the patient's family.

RECEPTIVE. In receptive aphasia the problem becomes evident when he fails to understand what others are trying to communicate to him. He no longer has the ability to recognize objects and lacks complete comprehension.

EXPRESSIVE-RECEPTIVE. The patient with expressive-receptive aphasia will have difficulty speaking and understanding speech, writing, and reading. A complete loss in all of these language skills is termed global aphasia.

The onset of aphasia is described by members of an aphasic patient's family in different ways. One family indicated that the patient began experiencing difficulty in speaking and noticed a weakness in the right arm, with a tendency to drop objects held in the right hand. Another family noted that the patient's speech became unintelligible and that he could no longer read or write. The loss of speech is evidenced by any or all of the following characteristics: (1) indistinct speech; (2) inability to talk; (3) distorted and incoherent speech; (4) difficulty in naming familiar objects, although their use is known; (5) difficulty in the use of proper words, alone or in context in a particular situation; and (6) difficulty in expressing ideas and thoughts.

DIAGNOSTIC ASPECTS

The language problems of the aphasic patient have been discussed in terms of interference with verbal communication. Different examination procedures are used to gain a better understanding of a patient's speech problems and to help evaluate his condition. The therapist may ask the patient questions and record his answers on an examination form. The patient may also be asked to point to objects, numbers, and letters, and to identify them verbally. He may be asked to read, to write, to count, and to feel different objects and to name them. While the patient's eyes are closed, he listens to a paragraph that is read and then answers questions about it. Eisenson's Examining for Aphasia Test, used for diagnostic purposes, consists of a number of subtests in different areas: (1) disturbance in the comprehension of recognized written symbols, (2) the loss of ability to recognize configurations normally received through sensory avenues, (3) writing disturbances, (4) arithmetic disturbances, and (5) spelling and nominal aphasia or anomia.

The diagnostic evaluation must be complete if the speech therapist is to define the level at which the patient's verbal communication is impaired. One should determine the area in which the patient needs training. The team treating the aphasic patient can plan the treatment program properly only with the information obtained from a complete speech evaluation.

SPEECH THERAPY FOR THE APHASIC PATIENT

In the ideal situation, the patient's condition should first be evaluated by a speech pathologist certified by the American Speech and Hearing Association. If the nursing-home personnel do not have recourse to a speech pathologist, they may look to the local medical center, rehabilitation center, or local university. These may provide the nurse with information on courses on this subject that she may attend. The nurse may also be able to observe speech-therapy sessions at the speech clinic and talk with speech specialists about the treatment procedures used in the total rehabilitation program.

Daily or weekly speech-therapy sessions may be conducted. The speech pathologist will instruct the personnel at the nursing home as well as the family of the patient regarding the language retraining program and the ways in which they can aid in the treatment program. It must be remembered, however, that where the services of a professional speech pathologist or therapist are unavailable, a great deal can still be done by the nursing-home personnel. If persistence and patience are used in an organized speech program, many of these aphasic patients can regain their ability to communicate. Booklets pertaining to aphasia are often used when the speech pathologist first meets the family or personnel that will be working with the patient. *Understanding Aphasia—A Guide for Family and Friends* by E. J. Taylor, published by the New York University-Bellevue Medical Center, is a helpful booklet, as are *Aphasia and the Family* and *Strokes—A Guide for the Family*, both available from the New York Heart Association.

Aphasic patients differ in their abilities and no attempt will be made to outline a specific therapy program. Berry and Eisenson have suggested that the materials as well as the approaches should be "tailor-made."

Considerable help may be obtained from certain literature regarding remedial education.

Initial Therapy. The most apparent personal
needs of the patient may serve as a guide for the initia-
tion of therapy. Words such as *nurse, doctor, food, water,* and *blanket* should be incorporated into the therapy
sessions. Exercises and drills should be planned around
the patient's interests, hobbies, and needs; this is most
important for successful aphasic therapy. The speech
therapist and the staff personnel involved in the treatment program should talk to the patient about things
within the level of his experience.

Sheehan has reported some of the techniques that
she has found useful in aphasic group therapy. Her
group used imitation, repetition, phonetic placement,
and such manipulation as coupling visual, auditory, and
motor images. The group capitalized on involuntary
speech and raised it to a voluntary level. Stress was
placed on speaking in normal phrases and sentences. It
was found that oft-repeated groups of words are said
as easily as a single word, and that they often promote
a rhythmic pattern of natural speech. Lessons were
planned about ideas based on units of work that were
a basic part of every individual's vocabulary. Emphasis
was placed on attempts to make the work as practical as
possible and to give the patient as many normal phrases
to speak as he could master.

The nurse working with the aphasic patient may ask
him to imitate her lip movements when she attempts
to teach the different sounds. The patient may acquire
a great deal of information from reading the nurse's
lips; for this reason, it is important for the patient to

be in a position where he can see the nurse. The nurse should have the patient watch the way her tongue moves when she is producing different sounds. It is good to have the patient stand or sit beside the nurse in front of a large mirror and try to imitate her tongue movements when he is trying to learn the correct manner of producing certain sounds.

A useful training technique is the coupling of auditory and visual aids. If the nurse is imaginative and creative, she can record different sounds around and outside of the nursing home on a tape recorder. She can also draw or find pictures of the objects that produce the sounds that she has recorded. For example, she may record the sound of a car or of a dog barking; then she may draw a picture of a car or a dog. When the patient hears the recording of a dog barking, he will point to the picture of the dog. Later, the nurse may record many different sounds and use different pictures; the patient is then required to match the correct picture with the appropriate sound—for example, a dog barking, a cat mewing, a horse neighing, a cow mooing, or a duck quacking.

If the aphasic patient has limited speech and needs practice in the area of better-connected speech and better comprehension, the nurse may use film strips in the treatment program. After the patient has viewed the film, he tries verbally to explain its content to the nurse. Story records may also be used in the same manner. If the patient is unable to speak, but can write, he may write out the content of the story film or record. The nurse may also plan a social hour, during which the patients are encouraged to meet together and discuss different activities in an informal environment. In this type of environment the patient may attempt more connected speech than in a formal speech-therapy session. The nurse may plan therapy sessions around the different activities the patient enjoys. If the patient likes to watch television, the nurse may have the patient watch a program and then tell her what the program was about and how he would have arranged it if he had been in charge of the production.

Some of the general techniques used with aphasic patients are mentioned to provide a brief overall view of certain therapeutic procedures. The following specific techniques are especially useful:

1. *Tongue-placement training.* Since apraxia of the tongue may be one of the most severe handicaps to many patients, drills for retraining the tongue in correct positions should be carried out.

2. *Movement of lips.* Lip-movement drills may be effective in helping to reduce apraxia of the mouth.

3. *Vowel sounds.* The correct production of vowel sounds should be initiated early in the treatment program.

4. *Consonants.* After the patient has learned to produce at least one vowel sound, consonant positions and sounds are taught concomitantly with the vowel.

5. *Syllable formation.* After the patient is able to produce a consonant and vowel, the next step involves combining the two sounds.

6. *Writing training.* Because of the close proximity in the cortex of the motor area for writing and speech, practice in writing the symbols while they are being spoken seems to help to establish engrams more firmly for both speech and writing functions.

7. *Building language associations.* Poor retention seems to be a strong characteristic of most aphasic patients;

their concepts should be strengthened through as many associations as possible.

8. *Vocabulary building.* To vary the procedures and to equip the patient with a useful vocabulary as soon as possible, groups of words may be presented in related units. Such units may be based on greetings, food, clothing, names of people, and parts of the body, but should include only those words that the patient is capable of producing with some degree of facility.

Berry and Eisenson call attention to the fact that both therapist and patient must be certain that the patient can understand what he hears. The therapist needs to make sure that the patient's response is appropriate to the situation. In the formal teaching situation, Schuell offers these suggestions for actions to be elicited from the patient: indicating objects in pictures presented by the therapist; executing directions; answering questions; completing sentences intentionally left incomplete; identifying specific words, phrases, or sentences that are spoken by the therapist (this can be accomplished by pointing, naming, or underlining); paraphrasing sentences spoken by the therapist; and writing answers to questions asked.

At times the aphasic patient may become frustrated because he cannot communicate verbally. His vocabularly may be limited to a few words, and he may attempt to use these words to express all of his desires. When the individual who is listening to the aphasic patient talk is not able to understand him, it may cause the patient to become frustrated. When the patient is unable to express himself verbally, he may want to write out his desires.

If the nurse working with the aphasic patient tries to force him to talk when he cannot or does not wish to talk, the patient may become depressed. If the nurse does not give the patient time to finish the sentences that he is attempting to produce, this can also be detrimental to the therapeutic program. Too often the nurse may not attempt to encourage the patient to talk and simply gives him objects when he points to them. Even when the patient is unable to name an object, but attempts to name it by making a sound, this may be better than just pointing and not uttering any sound. The patient might first utter the sound *wa* and then later say the word *water*. If the patient always gets what he desires by pointing and is not encouraged to speak, then the correction of his speech difficulties will be delayed.

If the speech pathologist or therapist wishes the patient to use a workbook, he should instruct the family and the nursing-home staff how to aid the patient with this type of therapy. In the *Manual for the Aphasic Patient* by Longerich, exercises are provided in which the patient can match words with pictures of objects, fill in the correct answers to questions presented in sentences, and provide appropriate answers to questions concerning paragraphs that have been read. The manual also provides other types of exercises in appropriate forms for patients at different stages of recovery. Another helpful workbook is *The Days at Home*, by Frieda Decker.

CASE REPORTS

An important part of the therapy program is the acceptance of the aphasic patient's condition by the staff. The following three cases illustrate three different types of environments and the patients' recovery program. These cases indicate the importance of daily communication, not only with the nursing staff, but also with visitors.

Case 1. A 65-year-old man, who lived with his sister, had a severe expressive aphasia, with only a mild receptive aphasia. After being discharged from the medical center, he went home to a very quiet household and occupied himself mainly by watching television and by reading news reports. His sister was counseled about the role she must play in his rehabilitation program, but it was evident that she regarded her brother as a burden. Although she promised that she would try to help her brother as much as possible with his language retraining program, she indicated that she had many community projects that would occupy most of her time. When the patient returned to the medical center a few weeks after being discharged, his condition had changed very little. Although he was now receiving speech therapy by a speech therapist in his sister's home, the therapist reported that most of the verbal communication the patient had was during their weekly therapy sessions, rather than with his sister. When the patient returned to the medical center for a check-up after approximately a year, it was noted that his verbal language ability had shown only a moderate degree of improvement.

Case 2. A 40-year-old housewife, who had suffered a stroke, had a severe expressive aphasia and a mild receptive aphasia. The patient's husband and her teenage daughter were greatly interested in the speech rehabilitation program and talked with the speech pathologist daily during the time the mother was in the hospital. The patient received speech therapy daily during her stay and returned to the medical center weekly as an outpatient after she was discharged. The husband and daughter provided a good speech carry-over program at home. When the patient's condition was reevaluated eight months later, a marked improvement was noticed, and she indicated that she now had only limited difficulty with verbal communication.

Case 3.   A 58-year-old man, who had been a foreman at a large company, had a severe expressive aphasia and a mild receptive aphasia. His wife and their two sons, both in their twenties, all worked with the patient in his speech rehabilitation program. The patient began receiving speech therapy shortly after the stroke, and the family helped daily. The sons included the father in their community activities and saw to it that he had a good opportunity to communicate verbally with other individuals. His wife received weekly counseling on the speech program and on the role the family could play in the total program. The patient received speech therapy weekly and made very satisfactory progress. After about a year the patient returned to the plant where he had worked before the stroke. He now had only a mild degree of speech difficulty.

The three cases summarized above illustrate the importance of favorable environment for the language retraining program and show how many people can cooperate in the program. They also illustrate how mismanagement of the patient can hinder speech rehabilitation.

The Laryngectomy Patient

A large number of patients undergo surgical removal of the larynx because of injury, cancer, or other disease. As a result of the complete removal of the larynx and a closure of the passageway from the pharynx to the trachea, a new airway to the trachea is made through an incision in the skin overlying it. A tube is then inserted through this opening, and air is inhaled and exhaled through the tube. The patient now must learn a new type of speech. This can be accomplished by expelling air contained in the esophagus through certain narrow openings that can vibrate; as a result of these vibrations, sounds are produced that can be molded into intelligible speech by the use of articulators such as the tongue, lips, and soft palate. Dunn has indicated that, for different reasons, approximately a third of the laryngectomy patients are unable to learn to produce effective speech by esophageal methods. For these patients an artificial larynx that produces vibrations is often utilized. The instrument is sometimes held against the neck, and in some cases a tube from the instrument is inserted into the mouth. The instrument produces sounds, and the patient uses his articulators to modify the sounds into words.

About 2000 laryngectomies are performed in the United States every year; it was estimated in 1961 that there were 15,000 laryngectomy patients in the United States. Local clubs have been organized for laryngectomy patients through the help of the state divisions of the American Cancer Society. Some of these clubs are known as "Lost Chord" clubs, "New Voice" clubs, and "Anamilo" clubs, which means, "We speak again." A number of laryngectomy cases are seen in nursing homes, and these individuals may want to affiliate with the "Lost Chord" clubs. A handy booklet for the patient with a laryngectomy and his family, as well as for the personnel that may be caring for him, is entitled *Your New Voice;* it can be obtained from the American Cancer Society.

Too often the treatment of those patients with speech defects has been overlooked. Such a loss of function presents a neurological problem that requires accurate diagnosis and definite therapy. A person who has suffered a fracture of the hip has an injury and function loss that is obvious. Loss of speech is no less serious. As nurses and staff members learn what can be done for these patients, their knowledge and experience will grow. As they acquaint themselves with the methods and techniques, their skill will become more proficient. The discussion in the preceding material should serve as a guide to the nursing home staff for more active programs in this field.

13

Recreation Therapy

I N the early days of chronic and convalescent nursing homes, the doctor and the nurse were the only persons concerned with the care of the chronic or elderly patient. The complexity of these institutions today has made it necessary for the medical and nursing staffs to become aware of related fields and to know how their services affect nursing and the patient. Nursing the aged is an application of nursing knowledge and other skills to the total needs of older people. The nurse must know the patient as an individual, not as a passing case.

The patient's needs can be satisfied with dignity and gentleness only if intelligent and understanding supervision is available. The elderly patient who is "unsupervised" by a trained medical staff often finds himself deluged with "untrained goodness." Institutional care of the aged is a failure unless it helps to ease their loneliness and offers them a real incentive to live. Medical and nursing staffs have come to realize that recreational service is as important to the individual as other medical procedures. A close and free exchange of experiences under the general supervision of a medical discipline is desirable.

Apathy leads to inactivity, and inactivity can lead to loss of function. Activity is a step in the reeducation of the patient. The concept of recreational activity has changed from frill to therapy; it should help the patient and give him a sense of achievement. It must be meaningful and not designed merely to fill time.

Where the quality of patient care is high, an organized recreational program with full staff participation is easily achieved. In planning a program, the recreational director works closely with the supervisor of nursing, who is in a strategic position to observe and evaluate each patient's physical status, needs, and capabilities. Her information can be utilized to the greatest advantage by the recreational director, who must understand the functional capacity of each patient—his background, education, and interests.

The recreational service program in a nursing home requires cooperative effort by the entire staff—by nurses, aides, and attendants. The supervisor of nursing, for example, may be able to arrange the time allotted to nursing care—that is, bed baths, treatments, etc. —so that patients can participate in the various programs. Sufficient time should be allotted before activities so that neither the patients nor the nursing staff will be rushed. Elderly people are slower and should not be hurried. The patients should be properly dressed to bolster their self-confidence. Care of incontinent patients is essential to avoid embarrassment. Each day the supervisor of nursing briefs the recreational director on the physical and emotional status of the patients.

The recreational director, on the other hand, must keep the nursing supervisor fully informed as to any planned activities. They both should meet all volunteers and assist in orienting them to nursing-home policies and procedures.

Objectives of Recreation

Recreation is defined by Webster as "refreshment of strength and spirit, diversion or a mode of diversion." Recreational activities take place during leisure time. Activities that are truly recreational must bring satisfaction and real enjoyment to the participant. A program of recreational therapy or gerontological activity must be offered, because recreation for the patient in the nursing home is vitally important. The patient who is alone, in an unfamiliar place, and concerned about his condition is uncertain and needs reassurance and a program of activity to help occupy his time.

This type of program must be approached with an open mind. It must not comprise merely so many hours of bingo, bean bag, and birthday parties each week. People cannot be poured into a preformed mold. The extent of the program should be determined by the patient's physical capabilities, his interests, and his past experiences. It should be the program director's objective to provide a suitable environment for his patient. People need to be productive; they also need to be with other people for "cracker barrel" conversation, and to be alone to "whittle shavings." An appreciation of the needs of the individual patient is vital.

The goal of recreational service as part of the rehabilitation process, therefore, is to assist in restoring the
patient to improved physical, emotional, and mental
health. One must be concerned with the kinds of recreational interests the patient can take with him if he
returns home, so that he has continuity of experience
wherever he is. Where return to the community is not
immediately feasible, recreational service should encourage the patient to take part in activity within his
capacity and to provide a social experience as nearly
normal as possible.

Some of the objectives of a recreational service for
the nursing-home patient are: (1) to offset empty hours,
monotony, and boredom and to help the patient adjust
to his illness; (2) to afford personal enjoyment and satisfaction and to improve morale; (3) to develop a feeling of usefulness and belonging, which strengthens a
patient's confidence in himself; (4) to relieve tensions
arising from mental, emotional, and physical strains;
(5) given added incentive, to renew and refresh physical
strength; (6) to develop skills, talents, and abilities;
(7) to stimulate desirable social relationships and promote sociability with fellow patients and staff; (8) to
develop awareness; (9) to enrich attitudes, interests, and
experiences; (10) to encourage creative, inventive, and
expressional efforts; and (11) to enable the patient to
explore vocational and cultural pursuits.

Minimum Total Recreation Area

Activities can be held anywhere if necessary, but, of
course, ideally space should be assigned for the pro-

gram. A room large enough to seat three quarters of the patients in the home for nonparticipative kinds of activities is recommended. This room must be adaptable; for example, it should be equipped with collapsible tables and chairs for table games or crafts and enough folding chairs for large groups attending parties, movies, or entertainment programs. This space should be completely flexible so that floor areas may be easily cleared for games such as bowling, horseracing, shuffleboard, or other active endeavors. The room should have plenty of windows that can be darkened for showing films; cabinet space should be available for items in daily use. The room should be equipped with adequate electrical outlets for a record player, tape recorder, television set, and a projector for motion pictures or colored slides, and good general lighting. The area should be bright, clean, and well ventilated and accessible to bathrooms and running water.

When possible, a separate craft room is desirable. In this way the many craft items with which patients work can be available at any time; such a hobby room that is accessible to use without disturbing other patients will increase these activities. It is advisable to have a recreational service office for the program director and space for storage of supplies.

Small living-type rooms where patients can quietly lounge, read, or visit are advantageous. Many homes have auditoriums, chapels, libraries, sewing rooms, kitchens, snack bars, swap shops, and small game rooms.

Such programs should also be concerned with developing outdoor activities. Paul Dudley White, who is recognized for his work in heart disease, has long championed the cause of regular, mild, outdoor exercise.

This cannot be overlooked in maintaining a well-functioning circulatory system. There is need to give more thought to outdoor walking areas and other outdoor pursuits within the capabilities of the patient. The outdoor area should provide a hardtop patio with easy access to the building. Walking areas are advisable for ambulatory patients. Chairs and settees and other outdoor lounge equipment should be provided. Space for lawn-bowling and croquet as well as shuffleboard courts is desirable for the summer months. Natural shaded areas or canopies are suggested for the patients' comfort.

Although not strictly recreational therapy, many patients derive much satisfaction when allowed to do certain minor jobs around the nursing home. Such jobs as sweeping the porches, wiping the outdoor furniture, pruning the flower gardens, and similar tasks may all be done by the more active ambulatory patients. These jobs can create a sense of purpose and usefulness that is often lacking in the geriatric patient.

Program Organization

Recreational activities must be designed for individuals who have special likes and dislikes, interests, and capabilities. In formulating a program, the recreational director is guided by the participants' hobbies, interests, and needs. Once these are determined, programs can be formulated, remembering the necessity for variety and the adaptability of old interests to present conditions.

A simple routine of time and place can be established

—for example, mornings for visits, afternoons for specific programs, and evenings for parties and movies. A program is successful in proportion to its preparation. The recreation room is ready, chairs are in place, supplies are at hand, the decorations are appropriate to the occasion, the volunteers have received their instructions, and the patients are expectant. The easy relaxed atmosphere, the congeniality, the apparent lack of confusion is created only by forethought. It is therefore wise to plan programs in time segments well in advance.

One should prepare at least one month ahead and allow three months for special activities. Thus, last-minute crises are avoided, budgets met, and expenditures made wisely. When planning any program, it is important to remember that it can be enjoyed three times—in *anticipation,* in *realization,* and in *retrospect.*

The anticipation can and should involve the patients in preactivity. This can be most effectively visualized by considering a special event. The program director meets with the patients, reminds them that the holiday season is approaching, and suggests a special party for the volunteers. A tea is decided upon, the date is set, the patients prepare the invitations for mailing, and work on the decorations begins. The planning group may suggest that each volunteer be presented with a small gift, so the program director shops for suitable items. Refreshments, serving, and entertainment are next in order. After a menu is selected, it is decided who will pour and how the tables will be arranged. There will be two shifts of pouring: Mrs. Jones and Mrs. Smith will handle the first half hour and Mrs. Brown and Mrs. Green the second. Mrs. O'Brien and Mrs. Clark will pass cookies. Someone must greet the guests at the door; Mr. Atkins and Mrs. Calahan volunteer for this. Mr. Cline will distribute the gifts. Mr. Edmonds will officially welcome the group and introduce the entertainment program. A recitation, a solo, and choral numbers by the entire group comprise the program; the rehearsals go on for several weeks. Mr. Hammond is responsible for the record player and the background music to be played while the guests are arriving.

For weeks this special program is anticipated and prepared for—all energies are directed toward the realization and excitement of the big day. Once the program is over, the memory of the good time and the fun of preparation lingers on, and plans are laid for even better occasions in the future.

TIMING

In the nursing home, programs must be scheduled during the hours of greatest leisure so that they do not conflict with necessary nursing care and medical treatment. Some individual activity can perhaps be conducted in the mornings after morning care has been completed. Afternoons generally comprise the greatest segment of free time and should be devoted to the major portion of group activities. In many homes, supper is served early; several free hours are then available for varied individual endeavors or special events. The utilization of all free time should be encouraged, with special emphasis on the afternoon hours.

Many homes prefer to keep weekends free of group activities because of family visits. In nursing homes located in isolated areas, however, the patients may find weekends lonely, and in such cases the director may make arrangements for special functions. When preparing for open houses or craft sales or picnics, occasional week ends are scheduled to involve families, friends, and other visitors. Holidays need special consideration also, as these may be especially difficult times for the patients. The entire staff joins in to lend a hand on these occasions.

PATIENT ADVISORY GROUPS

Once a program director has established rapport with the patients, consideration should be given to the formation of an advisory council, consultative group, or planning body. It is rare in a nursing home not to find a few patients who are capable and anxious to assist in every way possible. It is a pity to neglect the wealth of experience and knowledge that many of these people possess. Even a single volunteer can make a significant contribution. As this group grows in size, so does the response to any planned activity. This becomes their program and their ideas; they have a responsibility, not only to themselves, but also to others. They become the spokesmen for all the patients, and assist in determining their real needs.

One may sometimes be tempted to sacrifice the individual to satisfy the group; even the professional may become so concerned with meeting the needs of the largest number of patients that he forgets those of one or two. This is a serious mistake; the interests of the minority are as vital as those of the majority, and every effort should be made to satisfy both equally. An advisory group conversant with the interests of all the patients can suggest appropriate activities—for example, chess, stamp collecting, rug hooking, and carving—and can also implement these programs.

Program Content

Obviously, then, programs are determined by individual interests, routine is necessary, and activities are planned for the individual patient as well as for the group. This brings us to concern with the varieties of activities and their adaptability to the needs of the group or individual.

Myriads of activities, involving infinite variations, can be programmed for the nursing home. The success of any of these programs depends in great measure upon the leader, whether program director or volunteer, and the skill and enthusiasm with which he presents the programs and his ideas.

ARTS AND CRAFTS

Work in the arts and crafts stimulates interest and provides a real sense of accomplishment, for the result can be seen, handled, and admired. It is ideal to provide a display area for patients' arts and crafts where visitors, friends, and families can view the completed projects. Offering these items for sale can be an added stimulus; it can also provide funds for the purchase of additional supplies and materials. One of the patients can serve as clerk and run the store. Pricing at cost or just above cost on craft items ensures a quick turnover and encourages continued interest. Identification of the craftsman on the item by name can give a personal touch. Such recognition can be vitally important. Arts and crafts may be done both indoors and outdoors by bed-confined and ambulatory patients, as well as by the confused patient.

MUSIC

Music is an exceptionally good activity for patients. Group singing and the use of rhythm instruments are not confined to the ambulatory patient and provide spiritual uplift in every instance. Mimeographed song sheets with the words of old favorites can be prepared. Enlist the assistance of the patients to search their memories for the words of songs for mimeographing. Borrow song books for those not remembered and continuously add to the repertoire of old favorites. Search out the patient who plays the violin, piano, guitar, or other instrument and enlist his assistance for entertainment and for religious services or to accompany singing.

DRAMA

Skits, recitations, and pantomimes as part of a patient-produced entertainment program remain in the memories of both participants and audience. Storytelling and playlets can be effectively used when the patients devise their own story lines and plots.

FILMS

Probably the most effective program of this type is the slide program that can be taken to individual patient rooms for those who are bedridden. Travelogues, which can also be obtained in most communities free of charge, are very popular. Home movies and slides taken of patients in their activities are always greeted enthusiastically. Feature films, carefully selected, may be a monthly highlight.

Creating as near normal a life as possible in the nursing home includes provisions for spiritual fulfillment. Clergy and lay groups may be invited to lead meditation and rosary programs and more formal worship services. Bible readings and hymn singing lead in popularity. These volunteer groups may also become interested in personal visiting and in assisting with other types of activities. Many patients first become involved in recreational activity through participating in some type of group worship.

Special Interest Groups. Depending upon the individual interests of patients, many special programs may be scheduled. These may include gardening (window box or outdoor), cooking (where facilities permit), current events, lectures, discussion groups of various kinds, community service, fashions, collections of coins, stamps, buttons, and postcards, puppetry, and photography.

SPORTS AND GAMES
Unlimited possibilities can be envisioned for both the bedridden and the ambulatory patient. Adapted bowling, shuffleboard, croquet, horseshoes, toss games, horseracing, and bingo are a few. "Spare Time" bowling in a box is good for bedside use. Charades, quizzes, and guessing games such as Stop the Music, Name that Tune, Password, and What in the World? can be used by themselves or as part of another activity.

LITERATURE
A special-interest type of activity may involve book and play reviews, creative writing, and reading. A

nursing-home newspaper written by and for patients could include advance program information, staff news, ward news, previews or reviews of films, birthday announcements, new patient arrivals, patient poetry, a joke corner, riddles, and biographies of both patients and staff.

PARTIES AND SPECIAL EVENTS

These activities, requiring a good deal of preparation, involve the greatest numbers of patients. A monthly birthday party, celebrating each birthday occurring in that month, is a possibility. Halloween and Valentine's Day parties, a Fourth of July picnic or barbecue, a New Year's resolutions party, and celebrations of St. Patrick's Day, Christmas, Labor Day, and Washington's and Lincoln's birthdays are all opportunities for special activities. Talent and fashion shows, teas, bazaars, open house, and hobby shows can be scheduled periodically throughout the year. Trips and outings can be arranged in small groups by car or by bus when facilities are available.

Imagination and forethought are the prime ingredients of any program. Patients and staff of the nursing home may provide inspiration for untried activity; their active support in planning and preparation may be indispensable. There are few activities that cannot be adapted for use with patients.

Patient Motivation

To interest patients in taking part in activity requires concentration, imagination, and persistence. Even with such a captive group as is found in an institutional setting, the recreational experience must be voluntary—each patient must have the prerogative to make his own choice. The recreational director is responsible for arousing the interest required for participation. This requires an understanding of the reasons why some patients do not wish to participate. They may feel that their physical condition prevents them from participating. They may have a dislike of competition and fear failure. They may have a feeling of insecurity, rooted in loss of self-confidence or caused by a language barrier. Some patients may feel that play is childish, or may have ingrained feelings of superiority or inferiority. An occasional patient may resent enforced association with old or ill persons. Refusal to participate may be attributable to general dissatisfaction, the need to express independence, or inherent laziness. Many patients do not understand group programs and have been told that they are too old to learn. Friction among patients or between patients and staff members can also be responsible for nonparticipation. Frequently, a patient refuses to engage in group activity because he feels ashamed of his personal appearance or because he hesitates to reveal his physical disabilities.

An understanding of such factors is essential to the adoption of attitudes that will encourage participation. The suggestions that follow will prove helpful. Allow patients time to adjust; do not force them. Make sure they understand the program; involve them in planning. Acquaint them with the activity first by having them watch. Ask the patient to assist someone else; assure him he is needed. Use another patient to stimulate interest; arrange seating to be near a roommate or friend. Use a volunteer, a nurse, an administrator, or a family member to stimulate the patient. Ask the patient to be responsible for something—for example, as a reporter for the newspaper, to handle sales of craft items, or as a member of the welcoming committee. Help with an individual's special problems; help to improve personal appearance, if needed. Offer assurance or the opportunity to earn a little money through the sales of craft items. Suggest making something for someone in the family, for friends, or for a favorite staff member. Be positive in your approach—do not anticipate a refusal. Be sure to know the patient's background; find an activity specially suited to him. Above all, be patient yourself!

THE VOLUNTEER

It is generally impracticable or impossible to hire enough professional people to carry out a well-rounded activities program effectively. The volunteer is therefore the key to success or failure of a program. A volunteer is a person in the community who uses his leisure to provide for the leisure of others and actually participates in the recreational experience himself. The volunteer brings the community to the patient; he is the link with the outside world.

The volunteer becomes a friend, a source of constant enjoyment. He is an interested person, one who is reliable and whose visits can be looked forward to. It is the volunteer who assists with the craft instructions or writes letters for a patient. It is the volunteer who encourages and stimulates the pursuit of endeavor.

Recruiting Volunteers. This is both a difficult and a never-ending task. A director who is unfamiliar with a community can begin by contacting the local chamber of commerce to obtain a listing of all local organizations: church groups, civic organizations, service clubs such as Lions and Junior Chamber of Commerce, political and social groups, garden clubs, hobby and craft clubs, business and professional organizations, Senior Citizen's Associations, schools, libraries, Scouts, 4-H Clubs, YMCA and YWCA, and fraternal organizations. Every group is a potential source of volunteers. Persons who visit the nursing home may be approached. Appeals can be made through mass media such as newspapers, radio, and television. Volunteers who have become actively involved can supply leads to others who may be interested.

A telephone call to the president of an organization, with a brief explanation, may provide an introduction to possible volunteers in the group. An exhibit of items made by patients and a copy of the home's newspaper are valuable aids. Also helpful is a booklet listing the ways in which a volunteer may help; this should emphasize the flexibility of needs—insofar as possible, the hours should be arranged to fit the volunteer's schedule. Both skilled and unskilled help are needed. It is important to bear in mind the purpose of the organization being contacted; have specific suggestions that comport with their own interests and goals. For example, stress spiritual needs when speaking to a church group and display the kind of crafts that would be found at church bazaars and fairs. When speaking to teachers, look for projectionists and leaders for discussion groups or music and art appreciation.

One of the best ways to gather new volunteers is to put the most recently enrolled on the recruiting team.

They will be talking with neighbors and friends and will be able to channel a number of additional prospects, who in turn belong to different organizations that can be contacted.

Orientation and Training. Each volunteer should be interviewed and assigned a time of visit according to his needs and special interests. He either attends a group training period or receives individual instruction, or both. Organized volunteer training courses should be scheduled at least once yearly (more often when necessary) and may be used as a refresher course as well as for initial orientation.

Subjects that should be included in training are: (1) defining a nursing home and home for the aged; (2) understanding the patient and his special needs; (3) the goals and purposes of recreational service, including a general discussion of the philosophy of recreation; and (4) the responsibility of the volunteer. The training program should also include practical experience and instruction in arts and crafts, sports and games, music and parties, special activities, and bedside activities.

At the completion of the orientation program, a certificate may be awarded for those attending all sessions. For practical purposes the sessions may be scheduled one afternoon or one morning a week, for six to eight weeks.

Regimen. Volunteers report to the program director's office to check in and to receive equipment and instructions for each day. It is better to start the volunteer on the basis of one afternoon a week until he accustoms himself to the home; if he wishes, he may then be assigned more time. He is counseled that he must find a substitute and notify the program director if he cannot keep a commitment. Most volunteers are reliable, once they have made a commitment. They recognize that their visits are anticipated and appreciated by the patients.

A volunteer should understand that he may change his kind of service within the program whenever he wishes. He must also understand that he will be notified if the program director or the administrator feels that he is not suited for this type of volunteer service or if it is unsatisfactory to the volunteer or the patient.

Printed rules and regulations along with suggestions should be made available to the volunteer as part of his initial orientation.

Recognizing the Volunteer. The volunteer's value to the patient and to the recreational program is inestimable, but the volunteer himself must also be a recipient, a need of which he may be unaware. He must achieve some sense of enjoyment and satisfaction from having contributed his time wisely. It may be the satisfaction of doing something that is worthwhile; he may be developing a new skill or learning a new hobby and thus escapes to a new environment for a few hours. In any case, the contribution the volunteer makes is vitally important, and it is the responsibility of all to show their appreciation and respect. This appreciation can be shown by volunteer teas and parties given by patients and staff and by yearly awards. A simple "Thank you" can be very meaningful.

14
Selection of a Nursing Home

———•••———

T H E selection of a nursing home raises the question: What elements are present in the desirable nursing home that are wanting in others? The answer involves much more than the design of the physical plant, for the most modern and best-equipped institution is still only as good as the training, experience, and dedication of its staff. However, by indicating some of the check points that should be considered in the selection of a nursing home, we can try to point out some of the features that characterize a good, well-administered home.

If a person postpones the selection until a crisis develops, he will probably enter either the nursing home that has the vacant bed or one that does not meet his needs. Although an older person may never need a nursing home, he would be wise to acquaint himself with the various local homes and their services and facilities. This not only allows him to make a selection, when necessary, in an unhurried, objective manner, but also helps him avoid some of the mental trauma experienced by many older people when they are transferred to such a home.

A list of licensed and accredited nursing homes may be obtained from most state health or welfare departments. The Department of Health, Education, and Welfare, Washington, D.C., can furnish lists of nursing homes in the individual states. There is a distinction between full and provisional (temporary) licenses; the latter are usually given to the substandard home. Recently various medical, hospital, and nursing-home associations have agreed to accept the authority of the Joint Commission on Accreditation of Hospitals, which will set nationwide accreditation standards that will conform with federal legislation. Until recently, this authority was held by two opposing groups: The National Council for the Accreditation of Nursing Homes, sponsored by the American Medical Association and by the American Nursing Home Association, and the Hospital Association Committee on Approval of Special Health Facilities. Facilities accredited by these two groups will be accepted by the new approval body.

Further guidance may be obtained by consulting nursing-home patients or their families, the social service department in the local hospital, one's church (although in the minority, churches operate and maintain many excellent homes), and one's own physician. All of these sources may prove helpful in formulating a list of "good" homes, but in the final analysis it is the nursing home itself—its staff, its physical plant, and its atmosphere—that are the determining factors.

Location

When selecting a nursing home, a patient should choose one that is convenient for visiting by his relatives and friends. The more accessible they are, the more visits there will be. One should also remember that a central city location may be better for a city dweller who is used to the activity and the bustle of metropolitan life. On the other hand, some patients may prefer a suburban or rural setting. Although the building should not be in an area with heavy smoke concentration and excessive noise that would be detrimental to the patients' health, this does not necessarily exclude a city location. Actually, many of the best nursing homes are situated in or near heavily populated areas.

For homes located in the country, the availability of municipal piped water and sewers is advantageous. The average daily consumption of water for all services for each patient is 170 gallons per day. If the source and provision for disposal is less than this amount, it may interfere with cleanliness and good patient care.

Since over half the patients in such homes are ambulatory, sufficient level, graded, or paved outdoor areas suitable for walking and wheelchair use should be provided; this should comprise at least 100 square feet per patient. Out-of-door activity adapted to the patient's physical activity is beneficial to his physical and mental well-being and is highly recommended. Such space as a shaded sitting area for summer, a level lawn, and an area for shuffleboard, croquet, and a flower garden where the more active patients may participate should be considered an asset.

Physical Plant

A new building in itself does not guarantee a well-administered nursing home that provides good patient care; in the same context, an older building does not necessarily denote a poor home. In any case, the building, new or old, must be constructed so as to comply with the basic building codes, local and state fire codes, building exit codes, and public health codes. Zoning ordinances regulate the location and future building expansion of these homes, and approval must be obtained from the responsible authority.

SIZE

The present-day tendency is toward the larger nursing home. For example, there are plans for the construction of a 600-bed nursing home in Boston. Most experts agree that homes with less than 25 patients cannot provide the income necessary to offer skilled nursing care or to satisfy the new Medicare requirements. New homes today are beginning with 30 to 60 beds and with plans for expansion to 100 or more. If the homes are too large, however, they lose their home atmosphere and become too institutionalized. Although a one-story establishment is preferable for the smaller homes, obviously the larger facilities will be multistoried. The latter must have elevators large enough to accommodate either a stretcher or a hospital bed. In the multistory building, one should be sure that adequate fire escapes and exits are provided and conform to code regulations. The corridors should be at least 7 feet wide for easy moving of beds and wheelchairs. Since patients may be assisted by an attendant in walking, the wide corridor is highly desirable. All hallways should have grab rails and stairways should be provided with handrails.

PATIENT SPACE

Rooms. The patients' rooms should be on an outside wall, with minimum light equal to 10 per cent of the floor space and outside ventilation equal to 50 per cent of the required light space. A minimum of 100 square feet is recommended for single rooms and 80 square feet per patient for multiple occupancy—for example, 320 square feet for a 4-bed ward. Ceiling height should not be less than 8 feet, window stool height not over 3 feet, and door widths 3 feet, 8 inches.

No more than four beds should be placed in a room; however, single and double rooms have been found to be more practical and offer greater flexibility. Some physicians prefer to have patients placed with others so that the patient does not withdraw into his own world, but it must be remembered that on occasion all persons wish and need time to be alone; they also need a measure of privacy. Thus all rooms with more than one occupant should have curtains hung from ceiling tracks so that they can be drawn when a patient needs privacy. One should avoid all overcrowding.

The floors in the patients' rooms should be smooth and of moisture-resistant material that can be cleaned easily. There should be no doorsills; these impede wheelchairs and are a hazard to the ambulatory patient, who tends to trip easily.

Each patient should be provided with an adjustable hospital bed, an enclosed bedside stand, light, chair, and upright locker, 24 by 18 inches. Also, a call system from each bedside to the nurses' station should be provided so that each patient may obtain assistance speedily.

When visiting a nursing home, note whether patients are allowed any personal touches in their rooms. Are there family pictures on the bureau or personal possessions such as a favorite chair or table, a brush and comb set, or books? Such familiar things reassure these elderly patients in their new surroundings. Note also whether the patients are sitting in their rooms, looking bored, or whether they appear occupied and cheerful. When inspecting the patient area, note whether there are strong odors. Unpleasant or masking odors may mean that the incontinent patients are not receiving proper nursing care. These patients can often be retrained; if not, clothing and pads should be kept clean. Visible signs of dirt should, of course, be noted, but one's sense of smell is often better than one's vision in ferreting out uncleanliness.

Bathing Facilities. Many homes provide a water closet and lavatory for each single or double room, which is ideal for both the nurses and the patient. In any event, 1 water closet and lavatory should be accessible to the rooms of each 8 patients. There should be 1 tub or shower for each 15 patients, and 1 of each for each 30 patients. In multifloor buildings, toilet facilities must be available on each floor. Note bathroom odors.

Grab bars on the walls are a "must" in all toilet rooms to assist infirm patients to the toilet. They should also be placed in showers and tub baths. Showers should have the controls outside the stalls, so that water can be turned on from there; the stall should have a 3-foot-wide door and no curb, to permit the use of wheelchairs.

The hot water used by the patients should be thermo-statically controlled (the temperature should never exceed 110° F.). The floors should be slip-resistant, and rubber mats should be used in tubs to prevent slipping. A "free-standing" tub should be included. A call system in bathrooms is an excellent additional feature.

Other Patient Facilities. About 450 square feet of recreation area is required in a 30-bed institution, 600 square feet in a 60-bed institution, and 750 square feet in a 90-bed institution, excluding the lobby. There should be 10 square feet per patient for outdoor porches. Lounge and sitting areas offer a common meeting place for the residents and patients in the home. Patients must have space to move about and visit. One large lounge may double for a recreation area. Are tables set up for games, jigsaw puzzles, and similar activities, and are they in use? Passive activities such as watching TV are not as beneficial as joint projects shared by the patients.

In addition to the common lounge, small sitting or reading rooms should be included; again, these small lounges may double as dining areas. A central dining area for all ambulatory patients is an asset. Many state public-health regulations require that homes have planned menus; if so, does the food served match that listed on the menu? Does the home offer such special diets as low-salt and diabetic diets? Also, is the dining area clean and free of odors? Again, one should watch for overcrowding. There should be at least 225 square feet of sitting area in the dining room for each 30 patients.

Physical therapy and occupational therapy (work)

rooms should be available. Extensive equipment is not necessary, but full-time or part-time therapists are essential. An elaborate and expensive setup is of little value if it is not used, and used properly, with the guidance of trained personnel.

WORK AREAS

Depending on the size of the nursing home, a separate area should be designed for the business operation of the home. This includes purchasing, record keeping, billing, and filing of business records. In the larger homes, individual offices for bookkeeping and administrative services are provided.

The nurses' station is the control area for the supervision of patient care, and should occupy at least 100 square feet of space. A counter space of at least 8 linear feet of standard height and depth for charting and 10 additional feet of counter for work space, with a sink, small refrigerator for drugs, and an autoclave, are recommended. A locked medicine cabinet with adjustable shelves should be provided for the storage of prescription drugs. If there are over 60 beds in the home, it is recommended that there be a clean utility room of at least 80 square feet. The medicine storage area can then be included in this room.

Soiled articles must be cleaned in a separate utility room; this should be at least 8 by 9 feet for a 30-bed unit. If individual bedpans and urinals are not used, a bedpan sterilizer should be installed in this room. Soiled linen, bedpans and urinals should be stored separately from hypodermic syringes, sterile dressings, and medications. Since there is considerable soiled linen, ample space is needed. The soiled linen awaiting collection should be placed in covered hampers. Moisture-resistant floors and a hand sink are required.

A separate janitor's closet is recommended for each nursing unit, with a service sink and space for storage of mops, pails, and necessary housekeeping supplies. There should be a separate janitor's closet for the kitchen area. Again, floors should be moisture-resistant, and to a point above the splash line.

Separate locker rooms are necessary for men and women employees. This includes space for toilets, lavatories, and storage of outer garments. A small employees' dining room is recommended.

Kitchen Area. The kitchen should be centrally located and separated from soiled areas. The floor should be moistureproof, smooth, and easy to clean. Walls should be moistureproof to a point 4 feet above the floor. All equipment should be installed to permit thorough cleaning of the area around it. Ventilation should provide 10 air changes per hour, with screens on outside vents. Kitchen and dining room odors tell much about cleanliness and whether there is adequate ventilation.

Dishwashing machines are recommended, and the dishwashing area should be separated from the main kitchen by a 5-foot-high wall. There should be a 2-compartment sink for washing pots and pans, a vegetable sink for food preparation, and a handwashing sink. The cooking work center, which includes ranges, ovens, and tables, should have a minimum width of 9 feet. Garbage storage is in a fly-tight enclosure away from food-preparation areas. For refrigeration of food, 1.5 square feet per bed is recommended, with 6.4 square feet per bed for frozen-food storage. Space should be provided for storing dishes, glasses, silver, trays, and cooking utensils.

Laundry. The laundry service should have a domestic-type washer and dryer for patients' personal clothes. Since skin lesions are caused by irritating soaps, the use of mild soaps and care in laundering personal clothes can assist greatly in the prevention of ulcers and abrasions of the skin. It is optional whether sheets, pillowcases, and other flat work be done by commercial laundries or on the premises. Laundry and soiled-linen storage must be separate from food-preparation areas.

Conclusion

The nursing home is a home to the individual and should have areas and equipment for his care—whether he is bedridden, confined to a wheelchair, or ambulatory—and for his rehabilitation when this is possible. The physical plant may reflect the planning by the staff for the care of the patient, but the faces of the patients will reflect the warmth and consideration of the care given by the staff. The atmosphere is a vital factor in the ultimate success of any nursing-home program.

References and
Further Selected Reading

―――――◆•◆―――――

General

Conn, H. F. (Ed.). *Current Therapy*. Philadelphia: W. B. Saunders Co., revised annually.

De Reuck, A. V. S., and O'Connor, M. (Eds.). *Disorders of Language* (Ciba Foundation Symposium). Boston: Little, Brown and Co., 1964.

Di Palma, J. R. *Drill's Pharmacology in Medicine,* 3d ed. New York: McGraw-Hill Book Co., 1965.

Goodman, L. S., and Gilman, A. *The Pharmacological Basis of Therapeutics,* 3d ed. New York: Macmillan Co., 1965.

Homburger, F., and Bonner, C. D. *Medical Care and Rehabilitation of the Aged and Chronically Ill,* 2d ed. Boston: Little, Brown and Co., 1964.

Hooper, L., Mullen, D. G., and Kennedy, I. J. *Recreational Service.* Hartford: Connecticut State Department of Health, 1965.

219

Howell, T. H. *A Student's Guide to Geriatrics.* Springfield, Ill.: Charles C Thomas, Publisher, 1963.

Lewis, J. J. *An Introduction to Pharmacology,* 3d ed. Baltimore: Williams & Wilkins Co., 1964.

Modell, W. (Ed.). *Drugs of Choice 1964–1965.* St. Louis: C. V. Mosby Co., 1964.

Schlittler, E., Drucy, J., and Marxer, A. Antihypertensive agents. *Progress in Drug Research* 4:295, 1962.

Antibiotics

Barber, M., and Garrod, L. P. *Antibiotic and Chemotherapy.* Baltimore: Williams & Wilkins, 1963.

Feingold, D. S. Antimicrobial chemotherapeutic agents: The nature of their action and selective toxicity. *New England Journal of Medicine* 269:900 and 957, 1963.

Gale, E. F. Mechanism of action of antibiotics. *Pharmacological Reviews* 15:481, 1963.

Kirby, W. M. M., and Bulger, R. J. The new penicillins and cephalosporins. *Annual Review of Medicine* 15:393, 1964.

Diabetes Mellitus

Best, Charles H. *Selected Papers.* Toronto: University of Toronto Press, 1963.

Ciba Foundation. *Aetiology of Diabetes Mellitus and Its Complications.* Boston: Little, Brown and Co., 1964.

Marble, A., and Cahill, G. F. *Chemistry and Chemotherapy of Diabetes Mellitus.* Springfield, Ill.: Charles C Thomas, Publisher, 1962.

Heart Disease

Friedberg, C. K. *Diseases of the Heart,* 2d ed. Philadelphia: W. B. Saunders Co., 1956.

Luisada, A. A. (Ed.). *Cardiovascular Functions.* New York: McGraw-Hill Book Co., 1962.

Rushmer, R. F. *Cardiovascular Dynamics,* 2d ed. Philadelphia: W. B. Saunders Co., 1961.

Wood, P. *Diseases of the Heart and Circulation,* 2d ed. Philadephia: J. B. Lippincott Co., 1956.

Hypertension

Brest, A. N., and Moyer, J. H. *Hypertension: Recent Advances.* Philadelphia: Lea & Febiger, 1961.

Nutrition

Bogert, L. J. *Nutrition and Physical Fitness,* 7th ed. Philadelphia: W. B. Saunders Co., 1960.

Davidson, S., and Passmore, R. *Human Nutrition and Dietetics.* Baltimore: Williams & Wilkins Co., 1963.

Goodhart, R. S., and Wohl, M. G. *Manual of Clinical Nutrition.* Philadelphia: Lea & Febiger, 1964.

Mottram, V. H. *Human Nutrition,* 2d ed. Baltimore: Williams & Wilkins Co., 1963.

Wohl, M. G., and Goodhart, R. S. *Modern Nutrition in Health and Disease,* 3d ed. Philadelphia: Lea & Febiger, 1964.

Rehabilitation

American Medical Association. *Handbook of Physical Medicine and Rehabilitation*. New York: Blakiston Co., 1950.

Bierman, W., and Licht, S. *Physical Medicine in General Practice*. New York: Paul B. Hoeber, 1952.

Buchwald, E. *Physical Rehabilitation for Daily Living*. New York: McGraw-Hill Book Co., 1952.

Krusen, F. *Handbook of Physical Medicine and Rehabilitation*. W. B. Saunders Co., 1965.

Rusk, H. A. *Rehabilitation Medicine*. St. Louis: C. V. Mosby Co., 1958.

Psychiatry

Frank, J. D. *Persuasion and Healing: A Comparative Study of Psychotherapy*. Baltimore: Johns Hopkins Press, 1961.

Lowenthal, M. F. *Lives in Distress*. New York: Basic Books, Publishers, 1964.

Menninger, K. *The Human Mind*, 3d ed. New York: Alfred A. Knopf, 1959.

Post, F. *Clinical Psychiatry of Late Life*. New York: Pergamon Press, 1965.

Rochlin, G. *Griefs and Discontents: The Forces of Change*. Boston: Little, Brown and Co., 1965.

Stafford-Clark, D. *Psychiatry for Students*. New York: Grune & Stratton, 1964.

Sedatives, Hypnotics, and Tranquilizers

Domino, E. F. Human pharmacology of tranquilizing drugs. *Clinical Pharmacology and Therapeutics* 3:599, 1962.

Kety, S. K. (Ed.). Symposium: The pharmacology of psychotomimetic and psychotherapeutic drugs. *Annals of the New York Academy of Sciences* 66:417, 1957.

Remmen, E., Cohen, S., Ditman, K. S., and Frantz, J. R. *Psychochemotherapy: The Physician's Manual.* Los Angeles: Western Medical Publications, 1962.

Speech Therapy

Aphasia and the Family. New York: American Heart Association, 1965.

Berry, M. F., and Eisenson, J. *Speech Disorders.* New York: Appleton-Century-Crofts, 1956.

Carrell, J., and Tiffany, W. *Phonetics: Theory and Application to Speech Improvement.* New York: McGraw-Hill Book Co., 1960.

Corbin, M. Group speech therapy for motor aphasia and dysarthria. *Journal of Speech and Hearing Disorders* 16:21, 1951.

Dunn, H. A new transistorized artificial larynx. *New York State Journal of Medicine* 61:3463, 1961.

Eisenson, J. *Examining for Aphasia.* New York: The Psychological Corporation, 1954.

Gardner, W., and Harris, H. Aids and devices for laryngectomees. *Archives of Otolaryngology* 73:145, 1961.

Johnson, W., Brown, S., Curtis, J., Edney, C., and Keaster, J. *Speech Handicapped School Children,* rev. ed. New York: Harper & Brothers, 1956.

Kaplan, H.   *Anatomy and Physiology of Speech.* New York: McGraw-Hill Book Co., 1960.

Longerich, M.   *Manual for the Aphasia Patient.* New York: Macmillan Co., 1958.

Luchsinger, R., and Arnold, G.   *Voice-Speech-Language.* Belmont: Wadsworth Publishing Co., 1965.

Martin, H.   Rehabilitation of the laryngectomee. *Cancer* 16:823, 1963.

Miller, G.   *Language and Communication,* rev. ed. New York: McGraw-Hill Book Co., 1963.

Nichols, C., and Bressler, B.   A management program for severe psychophysiologic disorders: Anaclitic therapy. *North Carolina Medical Journal* 20:58, 1959.

The President's Commission on Heart Disease, Cancer, and Strokes.   *Report to the President: A National Program to Conquer Heart Disease, Cancer and Strokes.* Washington: U.S. Government Printing Office, Vol. I, 1964, Vol. II, 1965.

Ranney, J.   Laryngectomees and Esophageal Voice in the United States. *The Extinct Voices, Magazine of the National Federation of Laryngectomees.* Paris, France.

Ruch, F.   *Psychology and Life,* 5th ed. Chicago: Scott, Foresman and Co., 1958.

Russell, W.   Anatomical aspects of aphasia. *Scottish Medical Journal* 6:253, 1961.

Sheehan, U.   Rehabilitation of aphasics in an army hospital. *Journal of Speech and Hearing Disorders* 11:149, 1946.

Strokes—A Guide for the Family. New York: American Heart Association, 1964.

Taylor, M. *Understanding Aphasia—A Guide for Family and Friends.* New York: New York University Bellevue Center, 1958.

Wepman, J. *Recovery from Aphasia.* New York: Ronald Press Co., 1951.

West, R., Ansberry, M., and Carr, A. *The Rehabilitation of Speech,* 3d ed. New York: Harper & Row, 1957.

Index